"This book offers a remarkably easy way to get started and stay motivated. Just make the weekly appointments and Duf will walk you through the program. Now you can work out with my personal trainer, anytime, anywhere."
—*JoBeth Williams, client, actress*

"*My Personal Trainer* is a realistic guide to good health. Its common-sense approach helps you understand your body, so you can realize your personal best."
—*Andrea Martin, client, actress*

"The variety in Duf's program is a plus. Each weekly appointment offers something new and interesting. My wife, Susan, and I love the challenge of exercising together with *My Personal Trainer*."
—*Terry Christensen, client,*
Managing Partner, Christensen, White Law Firm,
Member, Board of Directors, MGM GRAND

"I've been following Duf's program for over 7 years. He gently guided me through two pregnancies while I worked a high-stress job. *My Personal Trainer* makes it easy for me to find the time to take care of my body."
—*Elizabeth Cantillion, client,*
Executive Vice President, Turner Feature Animation

My Personal Trainer

An Easy, One-on-One Approach to
Become Active and Feel Better from One of
Hollywood's Top Health Fitness Trainers

John Duffy
and
Megan Williams

CHRONIMED
PUBLISHING

My Personal Trainer: An Easy, One-on-One Approach to Become Active and Feel Better from One of Hollywood's Top Health Fitness Trainers © 1996 by John Duffy and Megan Williams

Library of Congress Cataloging-in-Publication Data

My personal trainer: an easy, one-on-one approach to become active and feel better from one of hollywood's top health fitness trainers / John Duffy and Megan Williams

p. cm.

Includes index
ISBN 1-56561-088-1; $11.95

Editor: Jeff Braun
Cover Design: Nancy Nies
Graphic Concept: Chadric Humphreys
Cover Photography: Thoen & Associates
Exercise Photography: Anthony Butala
Cartoons: Kevin O'Hara
Text Design & Production: David Enyeart
Production Manager: Claire Lewis
Printed in the United States of America

Published by
Chronimed Publishing
P.O. Box 59032
Minneapolis, MN 55459-9686

10   9   8   7   6   5   4   3   2   1

Contents

for
Patricia Duffy and Gladys Williams

We wish to thank Caitlin and Jacob Shamberg, John P. Duffy, Meg Kasdan, Esther Margolis, Lynn Preiss, Jody Sibert, Bill Delaney, and Diane Welhouse for their guidance and support.

Preface

If you think a personal trainer is a celebrity, rich-folk indulgence, consider this: the average American walks less than 5 blocks a year. And it's no wonder. After all, we have elevators and escalators instead of stairs; drive-through banks, car washes, and fast-food joints; automatic garage door openers and remote control TV; even CD-ROM sports! You get the picture.

It just may be that the technological revolution conspires against our physical well-being. Many of us hardly need to move a muscle to get through the day. Of course, we all know that over the long run, a sedentary lifestyle is hazardous to the health. So what's a body to do?

If you're like most of us, you need a hand getting out the door. That's where a good personal trainer, like John Duffy, steps in.

Duf's program is unique. The appointments are varied based on how the human body works. Duf not only gets you moving, he makes it interesting, informative, and fun. Best of all, training with Duf is like learning to ride a bike. You don't forget how to do it. The stretches, the exercises, the tips, and trivia are a lifelong good health resource.

So, that's why John Duffy and I wrote this book. We want you to experience the benefits of *My Personal Trainer.*

Megan Williams
Pacific Palisades, California

GETTING ACQUAINTED

Hi there! I'm your new personal trainer. Call me Duf and make me your close companion. Together, over the next 6 months, we'll change the way you treat your body—for the rest of your life. Now, that's a bold statement. But I know it's possible because over the past 10 years, I've helped many people reclaim their bodies—people like you who need a hand getting out the door.

I've written this book as a friendly, commonsense health guide. And, I've designed it to be an interactive experience so you, too, can enjoy the many benefits of a personal trainer. As your guide, it's my job to put you back in touch with your physical self. Along the way, I'll try to make sense of the health class textbook stuff on how the body works. I'll examine your eating habits and suggest realistic, healthy ideas for natural weight control. Most important, you'll learn to listen to your body, an essential technique that leads to self-motivation and confidence.

My Personal Goals

Now, since you're a new client, I need to know what you want from this program. Think about it! Please write down three goals you would like to achieve.

1 _feeling well_

2 _feeling proactive_

3 _longevity_

Take a close look at what you have written. No matter how you slice it, to achieve these things, you need to take care of your one and only body. The body that enables you to laugh, cry, swim, climb trees, watch TV, eat chocolate cake, dance, talk—whatever. You can't trade in your body, but you can take care of it.

With this in mind, take a moment to consider how you've treated your body over the past 6 months:

- How often were you involved in physical activity?

- How did you eat?

- How much rest did you get?

In other words, have you been practicing good health?

- The first good health practice is to exercise regularly;

- the second is to eat healthfully; and

- the third is to get plenty of rest.

It's that simple. From now on, these are the three things we're going to practice.

Chances are you'll slip up. After all, we are all human and are bound to skip exercise, eat a pint of ice cream, or stay up late. No problem. This is why I like to call it *practicing*.

We sometimes forget that achievements like playing the piano or learning to drive require lots of practice. So, to achieve the goals you've listed, you need to practice good health.

With practice, you'll look good, feel great, think better, and who knows, maybe add a few years to your life.

Whatever your excuses have been in the past, forget them! Make a commitment to practice good health for the next 6 months. If it helps, get a friend or your husband or wife to make the commitment with you.

Let's Get Started

All right, already! Here's how you use me. At the beginning of each week schedule three exercise appointments. Let's say, for example, you choose Monday, Wednesday, and Friday at 5 p.m. Write it down on the calendar page provided for you so we both know when we're meeting.

Then, all you need to do is show up at the scheduled time ready to exercise and I'll be there with the agenda.

One final request while we're getting acquainted; it will take less than 5 minutes and it's very important. I want you to put me down and walk outside to the front curb. I'm serious. I want you to put on some shoes and walk to the front curb. No excuses. If it's raining, grab an umbrella. On your way there and back, focus on how it feels to move your body. Go for it. I'll be here when you get back.

That was easy, wasn't it? It was also a big step because it demonstrates that you can get out the door. And it gave you time to listen to your body.

Congratulations, you have just begun practicing good health.

I'll see you at our first appointment.

Your new personal trainer,

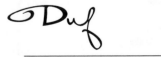

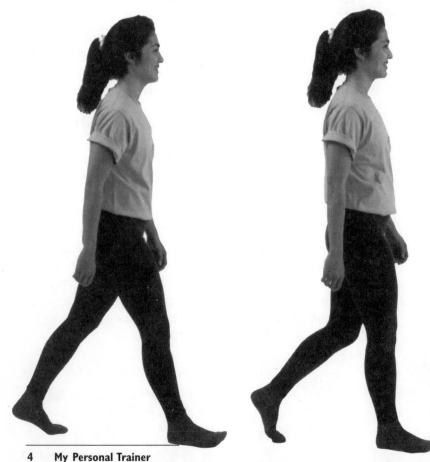

WALK

Left, right, left... or right, left, right. It makes no difference. Your body was designed to walk, so just do what comes naturally. Walking is a safe and effective aerobic exercise that helps control weight and tones the body. Most important, walking strengthens your heart—the key to healthful living.

Walking is a great opportunity to be alone and think, or to chat with a friend. Why not take the baby out for a stroll, and don't forget the pooch!

On foot, you'll notice things not seen from a speeding car. Maybe you'll happen upon a breathtaking view. Or stumble, I mean walk, across an intimate cafe. (Yum!) I do know one thing: it feels great to get outside and move.

Walking is fun and easy. You can walk anywhere—around the neighborhood, on a high school track, even in your backyard. Bad weather's no excuse. Just grab an umbrella or strap on some snowshoes. (Huh? Okay, how about mall walking?)

All you really need in addition to open space is a good pair of shoes and some comfortable clothes. When you have the opportunity, invest in a pair of walking shoes. As with any shoe purchase, first and foremost, listen to your feet. I recommend a shoe with a soft, thick heel. Why? Because when walking, you normally land on your heel first and good shock absorption alleviates unnecessary stress on the joints in your body (for example, knees, hips, low back).

Remember, when walking, it's important to keep the upper body warm. Grab a sweatshirt and if the temperature rises, tie it around your waist. Keep in mind a little sweat is beneficial. It regulates your temperature and helps rid your body of toxins.

Walking is the simplest and most natural cardiovascular exercise. Together, over the next 6 months, we're going to make walking the foundation of your "good health" program. So, slip on your shoes and we're out the door.

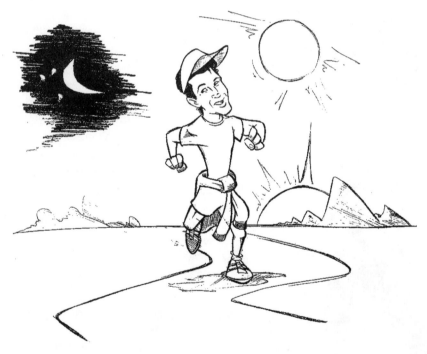

Morning, noon, or night, pick your best time
and schedule your appointments now!

Hi there… here we are. This first week, all I'm asking is that you get outside for three 20-minute walks. It'll be a piece of cake. Some of my clients choose to walk in the morning, others prefer the lunch hour, and some enjoy the evening.

Pick the best times for your three appointments and schedule them now. Write them down on the weekly appointment calendar.

Throughout the program, I will also ask you to do some light reading and writing. You'll learn a few things about how the body functions, enjoy interesting tidbits of trivia, and be able to proudly refer back to your accomplishments.

Oh yes, remember to examine each week's special assignment. It offers insightful ways to practice good health.

One final thought, as your personal trainer, it's my job to provide guidance. I tell all my clients that life is a long race. You're going to experience physical and emotional ups and downs along the road. No matter what, the goal is to consistently practice good health for life.

Okay, I'm fired up to work with you; so let's run through the drill once more:

•Schedule your appointments at the beginning of each week. WRITE THEM DOWN. If a conflict arises, no problem, reschedule.

• Do your best to complete each appointment as I've designed it.

• Practice good health.

It's that simple.
Let's go,

P.S. Hope you enjoy this week's trivia. Smile!

☑ Appointment #1

- Walk 20 minutes.
- Read "The S.A.I.D. Principle" (pg. 118).

☑ Appointment #2

- Walk 20 minutes.
- Read "The Matter of the Heart" section (pg. 119).
- Calculate your Resting Heart Rate (RHR) and write it on your Vital Statistics chart (pg. 117).

☑ Appointment #3

- Walk 20 minutes.

TRIVIA

Do you know it takes 72 facial muscles to frown and only 14 to smile? Keep smiling, it's easier.

Schedule your appointments now:

Monday	**Friday**
Tuesday	**Saturday**
Wednesday	**Sunday**
Thursday	*** SPECIAL *** **ASSIGNMENT** Fill out the "Self-Awareness Quiz" on page 143.

TRIVIA

Water!

Keep your body hydrated. Water comprises about 60 percent of your total body mass. Each day you lose about 2 liters of water through normal breathing and going to the bathroom. However, during strenuous activity you may lose an additional 1 or 2 liters of fluid per hour. Plus, smoking, alcohol, and caffeinated drinks dehydrate the body. Don't wait until you're thirsty; drink lots of water. I recommend having a glass first thing in the morning and just before bedtime. Remember: water is the source of life. Have a glass now!

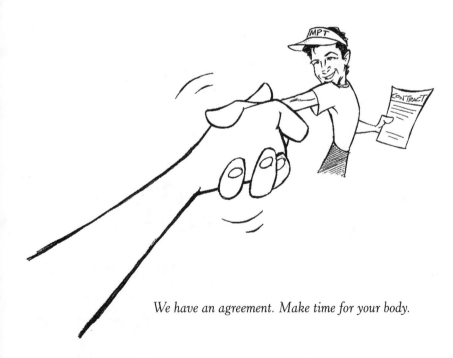

We have an agreement. Make time for your body.

Congratulations, you made it through the first week. I've found that during the first month, new clients often have difficulty keeping their appointments. Don't get discouraged; it's a normal trend. In fact, athletic clubs and gyms count on you to buy a membership, work out a couple of weeks, and then drop out. Not us! We have an agreement. It takes time to develop good habits.

My Personal Trainer is easy to follow and designed to require little of your time each week. Time is a major reason why many people fail at exercise. "I'm busy at work." "I have to drive my kids." "I don't have time to take care of my one and only body." I find these excuses hard to swallow, and so should you.

Think about it. There are 168 hours in the week. That's a lot of time. We're talking about spending 1 hour a week at first on your body and 3 hours a week by the end of our 6 months. I'll bet you'll enjoy the other 165 hours in the week a heck of a lot more. Remember, too, don't feel guilty if you miss an appointment, just reschedule.

Keep practicing,

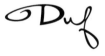

☑ Appointment #1

- ◆ Walk 20 minutes.

- ◆ Calculate your Maximum Heart Rate (MAX HR). (Refer to "The Matter of the Heart" section [pg. 120]. Write it down on the Vital Statistics chart [pg. 117].)

☑ Appointment #2

- ◆ Walk 20 minutes.

- ◆ Bring a tennis ball, or something similar, to squeeze on the walk today. It's a great way to strengthen your forearms.

☑ Appointment #3

- ◆ Walk 20 minutes.

- ◆ What did you have for dinner last night? Write it down:

  Mexican Food _____

  _____

  _____

Did it taste good?   Yes/No

Was it good for you?   Yes/No   _in bodies_

Schedule your appointments now:

Monday	Friday
Tuesday	**Saturday**
Wednesday	**Sunday**
Thursday	

* SPECIAL *
ASSIGNMENT

Drink at least five 8-ounce glasses of
water every day this week.
Here's a tip: keep a bottle in your car.

TRIVIA

I Don't Think I Inhaled

You don't need to think to breathe. Why? When excess waste products (mainly carbon dioxide) build on your lung surface, regulators in your body tell your chest to contract automatically. This contraction forces the lungs to expel waste products— you're exhaling. Then, as you relax, fresh air rushes in, filling up your lungs—you're inhaling. Put 'em together and you're breathing.

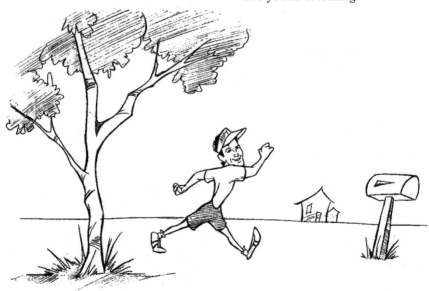

Pick up the pace. Challenge yourself with interval walking.

How ya doin'? Now that you're comfortable going outside and moving around, how about increasing the speed of your walks? This will help make your heart work a little harder. I've found a good way is to walk fast for short distances, better known as *interval walking.*

Interval walking is simply walking fast for a specific distance or time (an interval), slowing down to recover, then walking fast again. For example, I like to pick up the pace between two trees, or spot a mailbox up ahead and walk as hard as I can until I reach it. If you want to be more precise: walk fast for 10 seconds.

Your *recovery period* (the time it takes to catch your breath) during interval walking is a good indicator of your fitness. As you become more fit, your recovery period shortens. Your body is functioning more efficiently at work, rest, or play.

When interval walking, it's important that you listen to your body. Explore a little at a time. Don't be afraid to slow down if you don't feel right. By the same token, increase the number and/or intensity of the intervals if you can. Everyone is different, so you need to figure out your own limitations. I hope you enjoy the challenge of interval walking.

Hit the path,

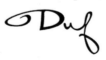

☐ **Appointment #1**

- ◆ Walk 25 minutes.

- ◆ CHALLENGE yourself with Interval Walking. Speed up for a few seconds, then return to your initial pace. Do 2 intervals today.

- ◆ Calculate your Target Heart Rate (THR). "The Matter of the Heart" section (pg. 121) tells you how. Write it down on your Vital Statistics chart (pg. 117).

☑ **Appointment #2**

- ◆ Walk 25 minutes.

- ◆ Read the "Breathing" section (pg. 122).

☐ **Appointment #3**

- ◆ Walk 25 + 5 minutes = 30 minutes.

- ◆ Do at least 2 intervals. Take a few deep breaths along the way.

Schedule your appointments now:

Monday	**Friday**
Tuesday	**Saturday**
Wednesday	**Sunday**
Thursday	

★ SPECIAL ★ ASSIGNMENT

Do you feel any different since we started the program? Write down two changes you've noticed:

none hardly

TRIVIA

Today is the First Day of the Rest of Your Life

Do you realize your decision to exercise may extend your life? According to a study in the *Journal of the American Medical Association,* a half-hour walk once a day helps protect against cardiovascular disease, cancer, and a wide range of other causes of death. People who exercise just a little bit tend to live longer.

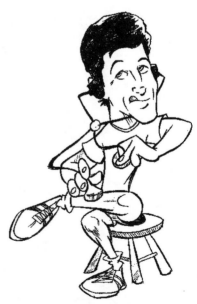

Listen to your body.

Alright!

You should be proud of yourself for making it this far. Have you noticed any positive results? For example, how's your energy level? Have you been sleeping more soundly? What are you eating these days? Remember, it's very important to listen to your body. I hope you're hearing a few good things.

This week we will focus on stretching. It's an excellent way to listen to your body. Are any of your muscles tight? I've selected 10 stretches which, when done in sequence, cover all the major muscle groups.

It will take some time to become familiar with the stretches, so be sure to refer to them often until you have mastered the routine outlined in the Stretching section.

Have a great week,

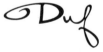

P.S. Hopefully, you haven't been tempted to skip your walks. If you miss, don't feel guilty or quit. Keep practicing! The days you really don't want to keep your appointments are the days you'll find most rewarding when you do!

☑ Appointment #1

- ◆ Walk 25 minutes.

- ◆ Bring a tennis ball to squeeze for some forearm work.

- ◆ CHALLENGE: Include 3 intervals in today's walk—make yourself work hard. See page 15 to refresh your memory.

- ◆ Review the "Stretching" section (pg. 124). Give them a try!

☑ Appointment #2

- ◆ Walk 25 minutes.

- ◆ CHALLENGE yourself with a more difficult walk today by using stairs, hills, or—you should be so lucky—walking barefoot in the sand.

- ◆ Bring a tennis ball and squeeze.

- ◆ Review the stretches. Try them again.

☑ Appointment #3

- ◆ Walk 25 minutes—pick up the pace and cover more ground.

- ◆ Bring the tennis ball.

- ◆ I want you to try all 10 stretches after your walk. Remember, static stretches are the best. No bouncing!

Schedule your appointments now:

Monday	**Friday**
Tuesday	**Saturday**
Wednesday	**Sunday**
Thursday	*** SPECIAL * ASSIGNMENT** This week, take extra care of your mouth. Brush your gums, teeth, and tongue thoroughly. Use a little dental floss, too. Smile!

SIT UP

This month we're adding sit-ups to our routine. Sit-ups are great for toning your stomach (abdominal) muscles. Strong abdominal muscles are important for good posture and help with digestion of food. They also prevent or assist in rehabilitating back trouble. Do the sit-ups before you walk, you'll find them a good warm-up exercise.

And, hey, don't be afraid to do a few extra if they get too easy. I've found that the stomach muscles get stronger a little more quickly than the body's other muscle areas. Sit-ups may seem tough at first, but stick with them and you'll be delighted with the fast results.

Okay, let's do a sit-up. Lie down on your back with both knees fully bent, feet flat on the floor, and hands interlocked behind your head. Now, keep your lower back on the floor, tighten your stomach muscles, and raise your shoulder blades off the ground. Do not pull with your arms, rather rely solely on your stomach for the lift. And keep breathing. I've found this type of sit-up to be the safest because it eliminates stress on the lower back.

Don't be disappointed if at first you can't get your shoulders off the ground. Keep trying! (That's one) Keep trying! (Two) Keep trying! (Three) It takes practice, just like anything else.

When doing sit-ups or any other exercises, be sure to maintain good form. For example, I'm going to start you off with 10 sit-ups. If you can do all 10 without rest, great. However, if you need to rest between sit-ups to maintain proper form, then do so. As your abdominals become stronger, you'll be able to lift higher and will need less rest. Whether you need rest or not, the goal is to do the total number the right way!

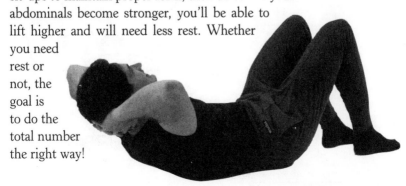

TRIVIA

Do you have any idea how long your intestinal (digestive) tract is? The average length for an adult is taller than a one-story building, or about 15 feet. Make sure you chew your food completely so the nutrients can be absorbed.

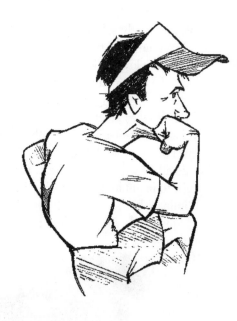

Think about it. How do you eat?

Hi there! I have a question. How do you eat? No, I don't mean, "Gee, Duf, I pick up my fork and stick it in my mouth..." What I'm asking is *how?* How often and how much do you eat?

Since exercise is becoming a part of your life, this month is a good time to focus on eating. Don't worry, though, we're not going to stuff ourselves with diet information. Over the next 4 weeks, we're going to consume sensibly, morsel by morsel. I'm going to serve up suggestions that have helped my clients and toss a few myths down the disposal. For instance, three meals a day? NOT! I prefer to eat lightly, more often. This helps fuel the body efficiently.

This week, let's explore *how* you eat. Nutrition will come later and weight loss will come naturally.

After much contemplation, I've decided the best way is to demonstrate some choices. So, maestro, a little music please, step into Duf's Cantina and check out the menu (read "Duf's Cantina" section pg. 130).

Adios,

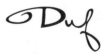

Appointment #1

- ◆ Do 10 sit-ups.

- ◆ Walk 25 minutes.

- ◆ Stretch.

Appointment #2

- ◆ Do 10 sit-ups.

- ◆ Walk 25 minutes—CHALLENGE—include a hill or stairs.

- ◆ Stretch.

Appointment #3

- ◆ Do 10 sit-ups + 10 extra = 20 sit-ups.

- ◆ Walk 25 minutes + 5 extra = 30 minutes. Include 3 intervals.

- ◆ Stretch.

- ◆ Check your Resting Heart Rate (RHR) and write it down on your Vital Statistics chart (pg. 117).

Schedule your appointments now:

Monday

Friday

Tuesday

Saturday

Wednesday

Sunday

Thursday

* SPECIAL *
ASSIGNMENT

Record everything you eat or
drink for three consecutive days
on page 148.

TRIVIA
Quick Quiz

How do you spell potato? Potatoes, pasta, whole grains, brown rice, and fruit are all excellent sources of carbohydrates. (Carbs should be 60 percent of your diet.)

Is the tomato a fruit or a vegetable? Tomatoes, bananas, and fruit juice (any clues?) are good replacement sources of magnesium and potassium—two important electrolytes lost through sweat.

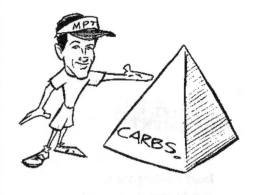

Make sure you get 60% carbohydrates,
25% fats, and 15% protein.

Gidday! Last week we focused on how to eat. This week, I want to focus on *what to eat.* The federal government has made my job a lot easier by creating the Food Pyramid (pg. 131), a graphic way to remember that a healthy diet is comprised of *60 percent* carbohydrates, *25 percent* fats, and *15 percent* protein.

Next time you sit down to a meal, take a look at your plate. Are the percentages in line with the Food Pyramid? Follow this simple guide, and your food choices will fall into place.

Eating healthful foods is one of our good health practices, so make it a priority to get healthy foods down the hatch first. Surely you remember "no dessert until you finish those carrots." I don't mean to preach but . . . you are what you eat.

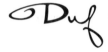

P.S. How are your sit-ups? Remember to use good form.

☑ Appointment #1

- ◆ Do 15 sit-ups.
- ◆ Walk 25 minutes.
- ◆ Stretch (Remember to breathe as you stretch).
- ◆ Read the "Shopping for Nutrition" section (pg. 131).

☑ Appointment #2

- ◆ Do 15 sit-ups.
- ◆ Walk 25 minutes + 5 extra = 30 minutes.
- ◆ Include 3 intervals in your walk.
- ◆ Bring a tennis ball for forearm work.
- ◆ Stretch.

☐ Appointment #3

- ◆ Do 20 sit-ups.
- ◆ Walk 25 minutes.
- ◆ Include 3 intervals, each longer than the previous time.
- ◆ Stretch.

Schedule your appointments now:

Monday	**Friday**
Tuesday	**Saturday**
Wednesday	**Sunday**
Thursday	*** SPECIAL * ASSIGNMENT**

Thursday

* SPECIAL * ASSIGNMENT

Let's go shopping. Read the "Shopping for Nutrition" section and draw up a grocery list for the week on page 134. Even if you don't normally do the shopping I want you to tag along.

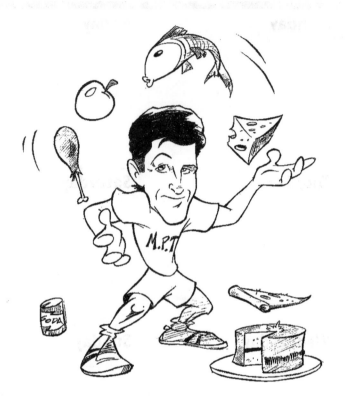

Duf's No-Fail-Guaranteed-
Natural-Weight-Loss-Diet Secret

The amount of calories consumed minus the amount of calories burned equals your weight gain or loss. Ta Dah! It's a miracle!

Seriously, a realistic weight loss goal is 1 pound per week. The only true way to accomplish this is to eat right and exercise. It's really that simple. Check out page 151 for an example.

Hi there! I was wondering if you know the definition of the word 'diet'? No, it isn't "a crazy scheme to shed pounds." Diet is defined as "food and drink considered in terms of its qualities, composition, and its effects on health." (Thank you, Random House.) Simply stated, your diet is everything you put into your mouth. Think about it. You can't go "on" or "off" a diet, but you can change it.

Thus far in the program, we've focused on how often, how much, and what foods we eat. Now, the stage is set to discuss *natural weight control*. If you want to drop a few pounds, you've already taken the first step—exercise. The only proven way to successfully lose weight and keep it off is to eat healthfully and exercise more. It's simple. If you consume more fuel (calories) than you burn, you will gain weight, and vice versa. The important thing is to examine the composition of the food consumed. After all, we're not going to put low-octane fuel loaded with artery clogging fat into a fine-tuned machine, are we? I think you get my drift.

Now, I'm not asking you to count calories or fat grams, but as you can see, weight loss depends in part on eating the right foods. Healthful eating combined with regular exercise will enable extra pounds to come off naturally. So, eat carefully and keep your appointments.

You're doing great,

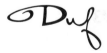

P.S. This week push yourself a little harder during the appointments. Remember, use your breathing to get through the challenges.

☐ Appointment #1

- ◆ Do 20 sit-ups + 5 extra = 25 sit-ups.

- ◆ Walk 25 minutes—CHALLENGE—find a hill and/or a flight of stairs. Remember to push yourself a little harder.

- ◆ Stretch.

- ◆ Describe your diet in one word: _____ (e.g., "yikes!").

- ◆ Read "Throw-Away-Your-Diet-Book Diet" section (pg. 135).

☐ Appointment #2

- ◆ Do 20 sit-ups.

- ◆ Walk 25 minutes. Explore a new route.

- ◆ Bring a tennis ball for a forearm squeeze.

- ◆ Stretch.

- ◆ Check yourself out in the mirror. What is your body type? What is your goal? (i.e., toning, strength, weight loss). Write it down in your vitals. While you're at it, have a laugh by making 10 funny faces.

☐ Appointment #3

- ◆ Do 20 sit-ups.

- ◆ Walk 25 minutes. Do five 30-second intervals (i.e., one 30-second interval every 5 minutes of your walk).

- ◆ Stretch.

Schedule your appointments now:

Monday	Friday
Tuesday	**Saturday**
Wednesday	**Sunday**
Thursday	

* SPECIAL *
ASSIGNMENT

Let's Do Lunch
Keep track of your lunches this week
(see page 152) and make each one a
healthy one.

TRIVIA

Out of Sight, Out of Mind

A great way to eliminate problem foods is to get them out of your home. When you want some ice cream, you'll think twice if it requires a special trip to the store!

TREAT

Duf's Shake

Fill a blender with ice and add:
- —your favorite fruit juice(s)
- —your favorite whole fruit (bananas, kiwi, peach, watermelon, etc.)
- —how about yogurt, raisins, or wheat germ?

If you like to experiment, try the shake (instead of milk) over natural cereal.

As they say in Southern California, wake up with a shake!!!

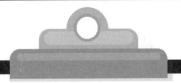

Okay, it's evaluation week. Our eighth week of practicing good health. Be honest with your answers! Write them down.

◆ Are you keeping regular appointments?　　**Yes/No**
　　—Walk with a companion and/or try new routes.
　　—Remember, I'm flexible; you can reschedule
　　if necessary.

◆ Are you paying attention to the foods you eat?　**Yes/No**
　　—Eat plenty of fresh fruits, vegetables, and nuts.
　　—Remember: 60% carbohydrates, 25% fats,
　　15% protein.

◆ Are you drinking enough H_2O?　　　**Yes/No**
　　—Drink at least five glasses per day.
　　—Keep a bottle in your car and a glass at your desk.

◆ Are you listening to your body?　　　**Yes/No**
　　—Beware of stress, emotions, and your
　　body's physical signs!
　　—Use your stretching time to listen and assess.

◆ Are you being challenged by the program?　**Yes/No**
　　I can challenge myself by _____
　　(i.e., more sit-ups).
　　—Include interval walking, hills, and stairs.
　　—Practice, practice, practice.

　　　　　Bye for now,

　　　　　Duf

☐ Appointment #1

- ◆ Do 20 sit-ups.

- ◆ Walk 25 minutes.

- ◆ Grab a tennis ball and bring it along on the walk. Squeeze.

- ◆ Stretch.

- ◆ Read the "Spot Reducing" section (pg. 137).

☐ Appointment #2

- ◆ Do 20 sit-ups + 5 extra = 25 sit-ups.

- ◆ Walk 25 minutes. Include 3 intervals.

- ◆ Stretch.

☐ Appointment #3

- ◆ Do 20 sit-ups + 10 extra! = 30 sit-ups.

- ◆ Walk 30 minutes.

- ◆ Stretch.

Schedule your appointments now:

Monday

Friday

Tuesday

Saturday

Wednesday

Sunday

Thursday

✳ SPECIAL ✳ ASSIGNMENT

- ◆ Let's do some housecleaning. Look in your pantry. Toss the junk food.
- ◆ Don't forget to check the freezer!
- ◆ Fill up your fruit basket and have a Duf's Shake for breakfast.

THE PUSH UP

This month we will work on strengthening and toning the back of the arms and the chest. The push-up is an excellent exercise for what I have in mind.

Grab the back of your arm (triceps). This is the biggest muscle group of your upper body. Next time you see somebody with muscular arms, compare their triceps to their biceps. Much bigger, eh? The triceps is a key muscle for any activities requiring the arm.

In addition, the push-up works the chest area near the armpits (pectorals). Strong pectorals enhance shoulder stability and contribute to your posture.

Many of us tend to store fat in the triceps and chest areas. Well, never fear, because the push-up is going to strengthen and tone both areas at the same time. It won't cause you to lose the fat, but it will help you get some shape. Remember, we can't spot reduce.

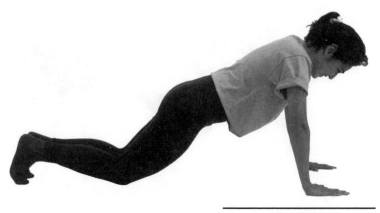

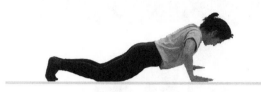

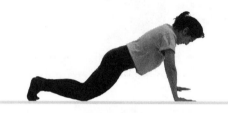

Knee push-ups

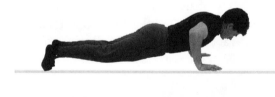

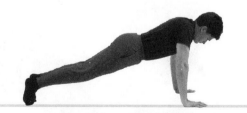

Regular push-ups

Okay, let's do a proper push-up. There are two kinds we'll be doing:

Knee push-ups—
The base of support is the hands and knees.

Regular push-ups—
The base of support is the hands and feet.

You can do either type, but regular push-ups add more weight to the exercise. I suggest starting with knee push-ups, then moving to regular push-ups.

Okay, we're ready. Lie down on your stomach with legs straight and toes curled under. Next, place your hands under the armpits with fingers pointing forward.

You're now in the proper position. Remember, for knee push-ups stay on the knees and hands; for regular push-ups stay on the toes and hands. Now, do just what the exercise is called and push up with your arms. Here comes the important part: When you push up, make sure there is no arch in your lower back. **Keep your back straight.** Once you've pushed yourself all the way up, slowly lower the chest toward the ground and lightly touch it, then immediately push up again so the arms are straight. Sounds easy, but it may take some time to be able to do one complete push-up. No problem. Work at it by trying to go further up and down each time. Your muscles respond to the work you place upon them (yep, the S.A.I.D. principle again).

Remember, if you feel an arch in the lower back, stop because you aren't doing the exercise correctly. Give it a rest, then continue.

Now, hit the deck and give me 20! Just kidding!

TRIVIA

Ever have trouble falling asleep? Try lying on your left side. You're using gravity to help blood return to your heart, thus reducing the work your heart has to do. You'll relax quicker if your heart is resting. Good night!

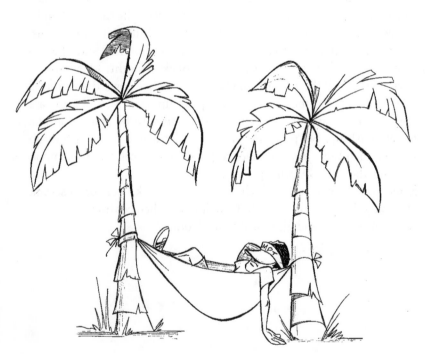

Practice your catnaps.

Hats off! You've now completed 2 months with your personal trainer (me!). You should feel darn good about what you've accomplished. So pat yourself on the back and keep up the great work.

Push-ups are one of my favorite exercises. I bet you'll notice and enjoy the increase in upper body strength by the end of this month.

Remember, when doing push-ups, *concentrate on proper technique.* Perform them slowly and take a breather if your back begins to sag.

This week we're also going to look at the amount of rest your body is getting. It is the third vital component of your "good health" program: exercise, nutrition, and rest.

Keep practicing,

Duf

P.S. Is the quality of the food you're putting in your body still improving? Remember, get the healthy food down the hatch first.

☐ **Appointment #1**

- ◆ Do 5 push-ups.
- ◆ Do 25 sit-ups.
- ◆ Walk for 30 minutes—include 3 intervals.
- ◆ Stretch.
- ◆ Read the "Rest" section (pg. 138).

☐ **Appointment #2**

- ◆ Do 5 push-ups.
- ◆ Do 25 sit-ups.
- ◆ Walk for 30 minutes—CHALLENGE—do a hill or stairs.
- ◆ Give the tennis ball a squeeze.
- ◆ Stretch.
- ◆ Take a catnap.

☐ **Appointment #3**

- ◆ Do 5 push-ups.
- ◆ Do 25 sit-ups.
- ◆ Walk 30 minutes—include two 1-minute intervals.
- ◆ Stretch.
- ◆ Calculate your Resting Heart Rate (RHR). Write it down on your vitals.
- ◆ Take a catnap.

Schedule your appointments now:

Monday

Friday

Tuesday

Saturday

Wednesday

Sunday

Thursday

* SPECIAL *
ASSIGNMENT

This week keep a sleep chart. How many hours are you getting each night? Write it down on page 155.

TRIVIA

Popeye was hip!

In addition to exercise, antioxidants such as vitamins E and C are thought to slow down the aging process. They help cleanse the body of deteriorating substances such as car exhaust, cigarette smoke, and fatty foods. Spinach is one good food containing both of these key vitamins.

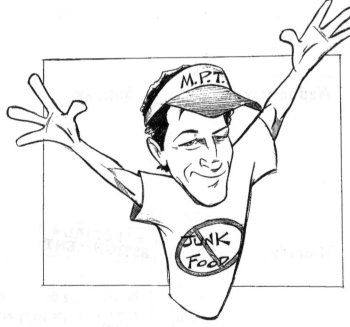

Give up one junk food for the week.
You can do it. It's only 7 days.

Okay, I haven't mentioned it, but you probably experienced some muscle soreness last week from the push-ups. No cause for alarm. Soreness is a natural result of the breakdown of muscle fibers and the lingering of waste products, such as lactic acid.

Remember the S.A.I.D principle? As you master the push-up, your body will respond to the challenge by strengthening its muscle fibers and removing waste products more efficiently. Thus, over time, there is less soreness.

You probably will experience a few minor aches, but most of my clients like the feeling of knowing their muscles have been working hard. *Listen to your muscles during each stretch.* Give them time to relax.

Bye,

Duf

P.S. By the way, how's your diet been lately? Just curious.

Dear Duf,
I hereby promise to refrain from eating the following junk food for one week:

_____.

Signed,

_____

☐ Appointment #1

- ◆ Do 7 push-ups.
- ◆ Do 25 sit-ups.
- ◆ Walk 30 minutes—pick up your pace by lengthening your stride.
- ◆ Put the squeeze on a tennis ball.
- ◆ Take time with your stretches.

☐ Appointment #2

- ◆ Do 7 push-ups.
- ◆ Do 25 sit-ups.
- ◆ Walk 30 minutes + 5 extra = 35 minutes.
- ◆ Stretch.
- ◆ Eat an extra piece of fruit today.
- ◆ Catnap.

☐ Appointment #3

- ◆ Do 7 push-ups + 3 = 10 push-ups.
- ◆ Do 25 sit-ups.
- ◆ Walk 30 minutes—include 3 intervals. Try to lengthen your strides again.
- ◆ Stretch.

Schedule your appointments now:

Monday

Friday

Tuesday

Saturday

Wednesday

Sunday

Thursday

* SPECIAL *
ASSIGNMENT

Let's make a small pact. Give up one junk (unhealthful) food for the week: cookies, candy, soda, coffee, chips, hamburgers, fries—your choice. Write it down on page 49.

TRIVIA
Avoid Traffic!

Hemoglobin, the blood cell that carries oxygen in your body, has 240 times the affinity for carbon monoxide as for oxygen. Carbon monoxide is a poison emitted by automobiles. You don't need it in your system. Pick your walking route carefully.

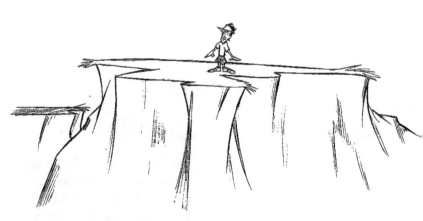

Have you reached a plateau?

How's it going?

With the exception of the push-ups, you've probably noticed your body has *reached a plateau.* Perhaps your weight and physical improvements have leveled off.

Don't be discouraged if changes aren't happening as rapidly as they did at the beginning of the program. I've found from experience that noticeable improvement occurs in stages. Be patient. If you are truly challenging yourself, I'm willing to bet you'll notice another change by the end of this month.

By the way, how did your junk food pact go? No matter what happened, keep practicing.

In fact, let's extend our pact for one more week! You can do it! Be strong! There's no need for garbage food.

Remember, a good way to avoid breaking down and eating that junk food is simply not to have it in the house. Get others in your house to sign the pact, too.

Have a good one,

P.S. Make sure your body is getting plenty of rest.

☐ Appointment #1

- ◆ Do 10 push-ups.
- ◆ Do 25 sit-ups.
- ◆ Walk 30 minutes.
- ◆ Stretch.

☐ Appointment #2

- ◆ Do 10 push-ups.
- ◆ Do 25 sit-ups.
- ◆ Walk 35 minutes.
- ◆ Put the squeeze on your forearms today. Grab a tennis ball.
- ◆ Stretch.

☐ Appointment #3

- ◆ Do 10 push-ups.
- ◆ Do 25 sit-ups + 5 = 30 sit-ups.
- ◆ Walk 35 minutes—lengthen your stride.
- ◆ Stretch.
- ◆ Thomas Edison did it regularly. Catnap, that is. How about you? Practice.

Schedule your appointments now:

Monday

Friday

Tuesday

Saturday

Wednesday

Sunday

Thursday

* SPECIAL *
ASSIGNMENT

◆ Extend your junk food pact for one more week. Initial here _____.
◆ Keep a sleep chart for the week. See page 155.

TRIVIA

Kick Up Your Feet

If you spend a lot of time sitting or standing during the day, be sure to periodically move around. Blood pooling in the legs can stretch the veins more than twice their normal size and lead to varicose veins. A little movement contracts the leg muscles, which helps the return of blood to your heart and prevents blood pooling. Protect your legs. Kick up your feet or stand up and stretch.

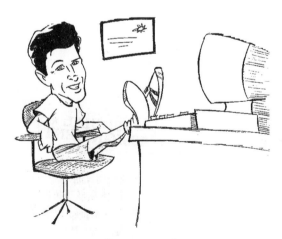

Protect your legs.

Hi! Hopefully, you have now adjusted to scheduling time for exercise. Have you found some days and times are consistently better than others? If you like to exercise in the morning, take a few extra minutes to warm up. Cold muscles are more prone to injury.

This week, let's learn another interesting fact about the body. As you will see, it's a great reason to *drink plenty of water!* Blood is the most important fluid in your body. The viscosity of your blood can vary depending on your hydration level. If you're dehydrated, your blood may become thicker. This makes it harder to perform its function of getting oxygen to all 45 trillion cells. Think about it. Water helps keep your blood flowing smoothly.

By the way, do you know how much blood you have in your body? Let's calculate:

Total blood volume is usually measured in liters. Just think about a 2-liter soda bottle to help you visualize.

Here's the formula:

Your weight _____ divided by 2 = _____ kg. times (x) .08 = _____ liters of blood in your body.

Write your blood volume down on your Vital Statistics chart and make sure to drink plenty of H_2O.

Have a super week,

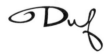

P.S. Next week I've got a special treat for you! No peeking!

☐ Appointment #1

- ◆ Do 7 push-ups.
- ◆ Do 20 sit-ups.
- ◆ Walk 25 minutes—CHALLENGE—you pick the challenge.
- ◆ Grab a tennis ball for some forearm work.
- ◆ Calculate your Blood Volume. Write it in your Vitals.
- ◆ Stretch.

☐ Appointment #2

- ◆ Do 7 push-ups + __? extra = __? you decide.
- ◆ Do 20 sit-ups + __? extra = __? it's up to you.
- ◆ Walk 30 minutes—include at least three 1-minute intervals.
- ◆ Bring the tennis ball along. Squeeze it!
- ◆ Stretch.

☐ Appointment #3

- ◆ Do 10 push-ups.
- ◆ Do 25 sit-ups.
- ◆ Walk 25 minutes—dig deep and do one interval every 5 minutes. Lengthen your stride—it's a great warm-up for next week!
- ◆ Stretch.

Schedule your appointments now:

Monday

Friday

Tuesday

Saturday

Wednesday

Sunday

Thursday

* SPECIAL *
ASSIGNMENT

Every night after dinner, go for a casual (5-minute) digestion stroll. This is a nice time to relax your mind. Check out the full moon...

LUNGE

This month, I'm adding my favorite exercise to our walking program: it's called the lunge. The lunge strengthens the entire leg and buttocks area, which leads to improved agility, balance, and stamina. Plus, it helps prevent injuries to the hips, knees, and ankles.

But wait, there's more! The lunge is the best way I know of to add shape to your leapers—post haste!

Okay, let's do a lunge…

Start from a standing position with both hands on the hips. Next, take a long stride, bending the forward leg to 90 degrees while keeping the back leg as straight as possible (the back heel will come off the ground). Lean the upper body forward with your head directly over the front knee. This keeps stress off the lower back.

Then, from this position, bring the back leg forward and stride into the next lunge. The idea is to keep stepping. Take long strides, one step after another.

Be careful not to arch your back (lean forward). Remember, as with all exercises, maintain good form. If you fatigue, take a rest, then continue.

Lunges require a lot of balance, so hold onto a wall or railing if you need to. Oh, yes, don't forget to breathe. We're working big muscles and they'll be screaming for oxygen.

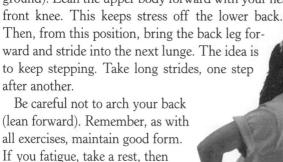

TRIVIA
Go With the Flow

Do you remember how much blood is in your body? Let's picture where it goes. At rest, the muscles in your body receive about 15 percent of your total blood flow, but during heavy exercise, they can get up to 75 percent!!! Keep moving.

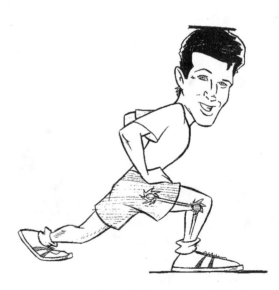

Love the lunge.

Hi there! I'm glad you're still with me.

The other day, one of my clients mentioned that learning to listen to his body has motivated him to stick with his personal trainer.

Think about it. We've accomplished a lot. You've just finished 3 months of exercise, sworn off junk food for 2 weeks, and learned a lot about how the body works. You're practicing good health. So, let's get fired up to tackle the next 3 months. Remember your commitment.

Okay, this month's exercise is the lunge. My clients love 'em because they immediately feel the muscles that are working. Remember, the lunge strengthens and tones the entire leg. It's a tough exercise, but the payoff is worth it.

Oh, yes, I didn't forget the treat for your body! Check out our first appointment.

Have a great week,

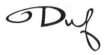

☐ Appointment #1

- ◆ Do 10 push-ups.
- ◆ Do 30 sit-ups.
- ◆ Do 5 lunges each leg during the walk.
- ◆ Walk 35 minutes.
- ◆ Stretch.
- ◆ Special treat: read the "Self-Massage" section (pg. 139).

☐ Appointment #2

- ◆ Do 10 push-ups + 5 extra = 15 push-ups.
- ◆ Do 30 sit-ups + 10 extra = 40 sit-ups.
- ◆ Do 5 lunges each leg during the walk.
- ◆ Walk 35 minutes.
- ◆ Stretch.

☐ Appointment #3

- ◆ Do 10 push-ups.
- ◆ Do 30 sit-ups.
- ◆ Do 5 lunges each leg during the walk.
- ◆ Walk 35 minutes.
- ◆ Bring along a tennis ball for the forearm squeeze.
- ◆ Stretch.
- ◆ Check your Resting Heart Rate (RHR). Write it down on the Vital Statistics chart. Any change?

Schedule your appointments now:

Monday	Friday
Tuesday	**Saturday**
Wednesday	**Sunday**
Thursday	

* SPECIAL *
ASSIGNMENT

Choose a rest day and schedule a 30-minute self-massage. Write it down as an extra appointment.

Blue Chip Health Tip

What investment will help you fight disease better than any drug, enable you to think more clearly, give you energy, increase your sex drive, help you sleep better, lengthen your lifespan, and cost you virtually nothing? Think about it… Exercise. Now there's a good deal!!!

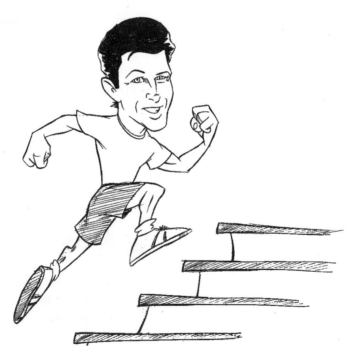

Challenge yourself and feel those muscles work.

Hi! How do your leapers feel after the lunges last week?

You should feel the muscles in the front part of your legs (quadriceps), the buttocks (gluteus maximus), backs of legs (hamstrings), and inner thighs (adductors).

This week I want you to *challenge yourself* during the walk. Try the lunges while going up a hill. Better yet, find some stairs. Instead of stepping on each stair, skip 1, 2, or even 3 stairs. Feel those muscles working now? If any of your muscles do get sore, remember, self-massage provides relief. Keep up the good work! And don't forget to smile! It's easy.

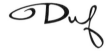

P.S. Have you been eating healthy foods? Review the Shopping for Nutrition section (pg. 131) and keep practicing.

☐ Appointment #1

- ◆ Do 10 push-ups.
- ◆ Do 30 sit-ups.
- ◆ Do 7 lunges each leg during the walk.
- ◆ Walk 35 minutes.
- ◆ Bring a tennis ball for your forearms.
- ◆ Stretch.
- ◆ Today, stand in front of the mirror and give yourself a 5-minute facial massage.

☐ Appointment #2

- ◆ Do 10 push-ups.
- ◆ Do 30 sit-ups.
- ◆ Do 7 lunges each leg.
- ◆ Walk 35 minutes—try 5 intervals of at least 1 minute each.
- ◆ Stretch.

☐ Appointment #3

- ◆ Do 10 push-ups + 5 = 15 push-ups.
- ◆ Do 30 sit-ups + 10 = 40 sit-ups.
- ◆ Do 7 lunges each leg.
- ◆ Walk 35 minutes—CHALLENGE—find a hill or a flight of stairs. Push yourself today, next week is going to be easier.
- ◆ Stretch.

Schedule your appointments now:

Monday

Friday

Tuesday

Saturday

Wednesday

Sunday

Thursday

* SPECIAL *
ASSIGNMENT Here's something
worth losing a
little sleep over. Wake up 10 minutes earlier than usual. Instead of getting up in a
hurry, lie in bed for those 10 minutes and
think. It will help you face the day more
relaxed. Try it every morning this week.

TRIVIA
Don't pee in the pool!

Ever jump into a cold pool and feel a sudden need to use the bathroom? When your body is exposed to cold, the arteries in your extremities constrict, forcing more blood into your body's core. This protects vital organs, such as your heart, by keeping them warm. However, your body's fluid regulators are tricked by this sudden increase in core volume. So, you need to use the bathroom. The body—a sophisticated system.

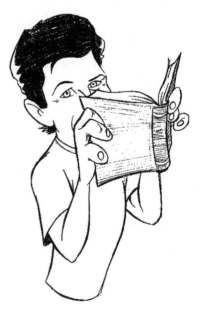

Concentrate on technique and communicate confidence.

¡Hola!

This week, let's ease up on the exercise throttle and *concentrate on technique.*

When doing the exercises, take your time and focus on your form. I want you to distinguish which body parts are working. For instance, pay attention to the backs of your arms and your chest during push-ups. (Just a little reminder to help you develop body awareness.)

Which reminds me to remind you about . . . hold it . . . don't move a muscle. How's your posture?

Chances are you're bent over *My Personal Trainer* in the all-too-familiar slouch. Pick me up to eye level. That should help straighten you out. Doesn't that feel better? Your vital organs feel better, too. Breathing and digestion can now function optimally.

This week, try to sit and stand up straight. Remember, posture is body language. *Communicate confidence.*

Stand proud,

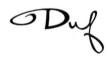

☐ Appointment #1

+ Do the exercises slowly and concentrate on your form.

+ Do 7 push-ups.

+ Do 20 sit-ups.

+ Do 7 lunges each leg during your walk.

+ Walk 30 minutes.

+ Stretch.

☐ Appointment #2

+ Do 10 push-ups.

+ Do 25 sit-ups.

+ Do 10 lunges each leg.

+ Take an easy 30-minute stroll. Your eyes need exercise, too.
  During your walk, practice looking at things in the distance. Read
  faraway signs. Can you spot a bird's nest? How about finding pic-
  tures in the clouds?

+ Stretch.

☐ Appointment #3

+ No exercises today!

+ Walk 30 minutes—pick it up; make it brisk!

+ Stretch. Do each of the 10 stretches slowly. Concentrate on your
  form. Massage the muscles while you stretch.

Schedule your appointments now:

Monday

Friday

Tuesday

Saturday

Wednesday

Sunday

Thursday

* SPECIAL * ASSIGNMENT

Here's a posture tip: Adjust your car's rear-view mirror while sitting up straight. The next time you can't see what's behind you, don't adjust your mirror, adjust your posture!

TRIVIA
Dem Bones

Your bones begin developing during the eighth week of embryonic life and complete their development around the 25th year. However, they are not as rigid as you may think. Bones are constantly being remolded according to the stresses put upon them. Exercise reshapes bones and forms tighter bonds with your muscles.

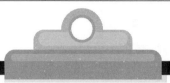

Guess what? *It's evaluation week again.* Believe it or not, this is our 16th week of practicing good health. Think about it. Four months. A third of the year. Wow!

Okay, be honest with your answers and write them down.

◆ Are you keeping your appointments?   **Yes/No**
  —If no, why not? _____
  —Just do it. (Original, eh?)

◆ Are you paying attention to the foods you eat?   **Yes/No**
  —How are you eating? _____ (one word)
  —You are what you eat.

◆ Are you getting plenty of rest   **Yes/No**
  —If no, why not? _____
  —It's your body's time to revitalize.

◆ Are you listening to your body?   **Yes/No**
  —What is your body telling you? _____
  —Practice body awareness.

◆ Are you drinking enough H_2O?   **Yes/No**
  —If no, why not? _____
  —Your body is 60 percent fluid.

◆ Are you challenging yourself?   **Yes/No**
  —If yes, how? _____
  —Nothing to it, but to do it!

◆ Are you practicing good health every day?   **Yes/No**
  —If no, how can you improve? _____
  —Keep practicing.

Now that you're finished, let's compare your answers with our first evaluation. Flip back to Month Two—Week Four (pg. 37). Any changes? This week, let's focus on the areas where you're having the most trouble. What will help you practice good health? Think about it.

See ya' next time,

☐ Appointment #1

- ◆ Do 10 push-ups.

- ◆ Do 35 sit-ups.

- ◆ Do 10 lunges each leg on your walk.

- ◆ Walk 35 minutes.

- ◆ Bring the tennis ball for your forearms.

- ◆ If you need a challenge, increase the numbers above. Write them down.

- ◆ Stretch.

☐ Appointment #2

- ◆ Do 10 push-ups.

- ◆ Do 35 sit-ups.

- ◆ Do 10 lunges each leg.

- ◆ Walk for 40 minutes. Guess what? You just doubled your walk time since you began this program. Congrats!

- ◆ Stretch.

☐ Appointment #3

- ◆ Remember junior high? Try 10 jumping jacks today. That'll get the blood pumping.

- ◆ Do 10 push-ups.

- ◆ Do 35 sit-ups.

- ◆ Do 10 lunges each leg.

- ◆ Walk 40 minutes.

- ◆ Stretch.

Schedule your appointments now:

Monday

Tuesday

Wednesday

Thursday

Friday

Saturday

Sunday

* SPECIAL *
ASSIGNMENT

I want you to eat absolutely no greasy foods this week. Yep, that includes french fries, and bacon, and ... you know the foods. It's my job to be strict once in a while.

CURLS

This month we will strengthen the front part of the arm (biceps) with the next exercise: the curl. We do curls all the time without being aware of it. Every time you pick something up—a glass of water, the car keys, this book, you name it—you are using your biceps muscle.

Now, let's try a curl: start in a standing position with feet shoulder width apart and knees slightly bent. Your arms should be hanging at your sides, palms facing forward. Look straight ahead and use perfect posture. Now, keep your elbows touching your sides, and bring your hands up toward their respective shoulders. After the hands are as high as they can go, s-l-o-w-l-y lower them back to your sides and you've done a complete curl! Piece of cake!

Although weights are not essential when doing curls, my clients use them for added resistance. I prefer light weights. For women I recommend 3 to 5 pounds, and for men 5 to 10 pounds. You can also use soup cans, rocks, or anything you can hold that has a little weight.

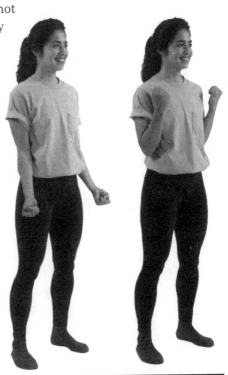

Without weights, you can create resistance by keeping the biceps tight both on the upward and downward motion of the curl. You can increase this resistance by clenching your fists tightly, which also benefits your forearms. Added resistance on the downward motion will work your triceps, too.

TRIVIA

SEXy

When was the last time you learned something new about sex? Your cells contain 46 chromosomes—22 pairs of non-sex chromosomes and one pair of sex chromosomes. Males have one X and one Y sex chromosome, while females have two X sex chromosomes. XY and XX—the only difference between men and women? Think about it.

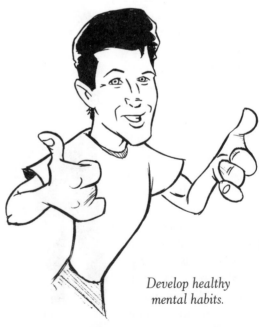

Develop healthy mental habits.

SEX. Now that I have your attention, don't flake out on me. You're close to making exercise a true part of your life. You're thinking about it these days, and if you skip an appointment, I bet you even miss it.

Now, before I tell you what's in store for you this week, I want you to take a couple of deep breaths, close your eyes, and try to remember a funny experience from your childhood. It's fun to daydream, and it's healthy to let your mind wander. Come on, think hard. There has to be one funny experience. Take a few minutes and laugh out loud.

This may seem irrelevant, but I really want you to try it. There is a relationship between emotional and physical well being, so it's important to develop healthful mental habits, too. Try to offset negativity by thinking kind and happy thoughts. With practice your outlook will become more positive and you'll feel healthier.

Okay. This week we've added curls to the program. After a few tries, I'm sure you'll find them easy.

Smile,

P.S. Check out the trivia for more on SEX!!!

☐ Appointment #1

- ◆ Do 10 curls.
- ◆ Do 10 push-ups.
- ◆ Do 30 sit-ups.
- ◆ Do 10 lunges on your walk.
- ◆ Walk 30 minutes. Include six 30-second intervals.
- ◆ Today, give yourself a facial massage under a nice warm shower!

☐ Appointment #2

- ◆ Do 10 curls.
- ◆ Do 10 push-ups.
- ◆ Do 35 sit-ups.
- ◆ Do 10 lunges on your walk.
- ◆ Walk 35 minutes. Let's do six more 30-second intervals.
- ◆ Give the tennis ball a squeeze.
- ◆ Stretch.
- ◆ Take a 10-minute catnap. Keep practicing.

☐ Appointment #3

- ◆ Do 10 curls.
- ◆ Do 10 push-ups.
- ◆ Do 35 sit-ups.
- ◆ Do 10 lunges on the walk.
- ◆ Check your RHR and mark it down on the Vital Statistics chart. Notice any difference?
- ◆ Walk 35 minutes.
- ◆ Stretch.

Schedule your appointments now:

Monday

Friday

Tuesday

Saturday

Wednesday

Sunday

Thursday

* SPECIAL *
ASSIGNMENT

Practice relaxing. Close your eyes and take a deep breath. Inhale completely. Hold it for a second. Exhale completely. Do 3 times. Relaxed? Next time you find yourself in a stressful situation, take a few deep breaths.

Supply and Demand

Ever get light-headed from exercise? If you stop exercising suddenly, your blood pressure drops, causing a dizzy feeling. This is because your heart continues to beat fast, but a lack of muscle contraction leads to less blood returning to your heart. This causes a momentary lapse of blood supply to the brain. After an exercise stint, keep the muscles contracting by moving around and/or stretching for at least 5 minutes.

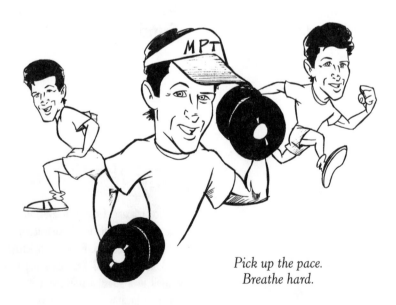

Pick up the pace.
Breathe hard.

Okay, let's get psyched up for *Duf's Tuf Week.* This week, I not only want you to push yourself, I want you to add a fourth appointment to your schedule.

Challenge yourself. *Pick up the pace.* Exert your body until you're breathing hard. Occasional, intense exercise can spice up a program. More importantly, it can advance your performance to a new level. How does this happen? Refresh your memory by re-reading the S.A.I.D. principle (pg. 118). When you work hard, your muscle fibers break down; during rest, they rebuild stronger than before.

As your personal trainer, I stagger the intensity and duration of exercise so your body gets gradually stronger without injury. You're already into your fifth month. Just think how you'll feel in a year!

Go get 'em,

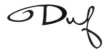

P.S. Focus on your body and use your mind to help push you that extra step.

P.P.S. Don't forget to drink plenty of water.

☐ Appointment #1

- ◆ Do 10 curls + 10 extra = 20 curls.
- ◆ Do 20 push-ups.
- ◆ Do 40 sit-ups.
- ◆ Do 15 lunges during the walk.
- ◆ Walk 40 minutes—do 5 intervals—push yourself!
- ◆ Take a tennis ball on your walk and do 10 curls while squeezing the ball.
- ◆ Stretch.

☐ Appointment #2

- ◆ Do 20 curls.
- ◆ Do 20 push-ups.
- ◆ Do 45 sit-ups.
- ◆ Do 15 lunges during the walk.
- ◆ Walk 40 minutes—do 5 intervals of at least 1 minute each.
- ◆ Check your heart rate before and after a brisk interval. Any difference?
- ◆ Stretch.

☐ Appointment #3

- ◆ Do 25 curls.
- ◆ Do 20 push-ups.
- ◆ Do 50 sit-ups.
- ◆ Do 20 lunges.
- ◆ Walk 40 minutes—do 5 intervals of at least 1 1/2 minutes each; try increasing the length of your stride.
- ◆ Stretch.
- ◆ Take an extra 10 minutes for a catnap today.

☐ Appointment #4

- ◆ Walk 45 minutes at a comfortable pace.
- ◆ Stretch for at least 15 minutes.

Schedule your appointments now:

Monday

Friday

Tuesday

Saturday

Wednesday

Sunday

Thursday

* SPECIAL *
ASSIGNMENT

Give yourself a 20-minute full-body massage. Schedule it now.
That makes five appointments this week. Great job!

TRIVIA

Ouch!!

If you ever get a cut, scrape, or scratch, wash it off and rub the natural gel of an aloe vera plant on the wound. I've found aloe vera helps speed recovery and reduces scarring.

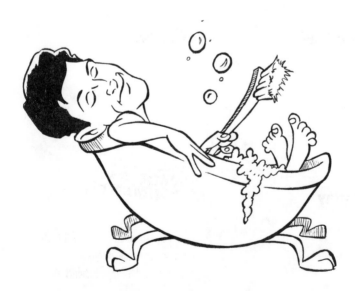

Grooming is another way to take care of your body.

Howdy! How'd it go last week? You worked hard. You kicked b___ (gluteus maximus). Didn't it feel great?

How about a *week at the spa?* You deserve it. Let's focus on cleaning your body. Grooming can be a pleasurable time to take special care of yourself. Take advantage of this opportunity to relax, unwind, and cleanse your soul, so to speak.

Your skin is the largest organ of your body. Don't smother it. Let it breathe! Be careful not to use harsh soaps, shampoos, deodorants, and toothpaste. Read the labels. These products are often abrasive and drying, causing more harm than good.

Unless you roll around in the dirt, you don't need to lather up every time you bathe. A little soap in strategic spots and lots of plain water will keep your body sufficiently clean and moist.

If you use oils or lotions, apply them *sparingly* while you're still wet. It's better for your skin, not to mention your wallet.

Now, open wide. Your mouth needs care, too. Brush your mouth thoroughly—teeth, gums, and tongue. Daily flossing eliminates food particles and helps keep your breath fresh. More importantly, flossing helps maintain strong teeth and gums. I just timed it. It took me 53 seconds to floss my teeth. Can you beat that?

Here are a few more suggestions:

♦ Alternating hot and cold water in the shower is invigorating.
♦ Dry brushing before bathing or a loofah scrub in the shower removes dead skin cells.
♦ Olive oil is a natural alternative to commercial lotions.
♦ Cucumber slices on the eyelids are soothing.

A clean you is a healthier you. Oh yeah . . . don't forget to clean your nails and wash behind your ears!

P.S. Use an all-natural toothpaste for the remainder of the month. It may take awhile to become accustomed to the change, but I'll bet your mouth will smile.

Thanks, Mom!

Duf

☐ Appointment #1

- ◆ Do 10 curls.
- ◆ Do 10 push-ups.
- ◆ Do 25 sit-ups.
- ◆ Do 10 lunges.
- ◆ Walk as fast as you can for 20 minutes.
- ◆ Stretch.
- ◆ This week, concentrate on correct form when doing the exercises.

☐ Appointment #2

- ◆ Do 15 curls.
- ◆ Do 15 push-ups.
- ◆ Do 30 sit-ups.
- ◆ Do 10 lunges.
- ◆ Walk 25 minutes—take a casual stroll.
- ◆ Bring a tennis ball for the grippers.
- ◆ Stretch.
- ◆ Invite a companion to join us on the next walk.

☐ Appointment #3

- ◆ Do 20 curls.
- ◆ Do 15 push-ups.
- ◆ Do 35 sit-ups.
- ◆ Do 15 lunges.
- ◆ Walk 30 minutes—do 5 intervals, each only 10 seconds long, as hard as you can—breathe.
- ◆ Have a great stretch—massage your muscles!

Schedule your appointments now:

Monday

Friday

Tuesday

Saturday

Wednesday

Sunday

Thursday

* SPECIAL *
ASSIGNMENT

Remember it's spa week. Take time for yourself. Brew a cup of tea, run a relaxing bath, and give yourself a massage. Schedule your break now. Enjoy!

Weekly Time Budget

Fixed Hours		Variable Hours	
Rest	_____	Errands	_____
Work (including your commute)	_____	Social life	_____
		Hobbies	_____
Meals	_____	Daydreaming	_____
Exercise	_____	Vacations	_____
Grooming	_____	Other	_____
Family time	_____	Significant other	_____

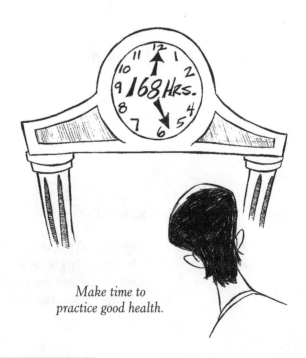

Make time to practice good health.

They say time is money, so let's take a look at how you budget. Not your finances—your time.

Think of fixed and variable categories. Fixed are those things that are essential, like rent, utilities, and car payments. Variables are discretionary expenses, such as clothes, movies, and hockey games.

This week, let's practice becoming aware of how you use your time and learn to respect the hours that you have—all 168 of 'em.

Okay, let's sit down and draw up a time budget. You can add or delete categories as needed.

You may be surprised how much time you do have to practice good health.

Gotta' walk,

Duf

P.S. Don't forget flossing time—53 seconds per day!

☐ Appointment #1

- ◆ Do 10 curls.
- ◆ Do 15 push-ups.
- ◆ Do 35 sit-ups.
- ◆ Do 10 lunges during the walk.
- ◆ Walk for 35 minutes—walk briskly. CHALLENGE yourself with a hill or some stairs.
- ◆ Stretch.

☐ Appointment #2

- ◆ Do 15 curls.
- ◆ Do 15 push-ups.
- ◆ Do 35 sit-ups.
- ◆ Do 10 lunges.
- ◆ Walk 35 minutes.
- ◆ Focus on proper form today.
- ◆ "Squeeze me," said the tennis ball.
- ◆ Stretch.

☐ Appointment #3

- ◆ Do 15 curls. Can you do all 15 without resting?
- ◆ Do 15 push-ups. Can you do all 15 without resting?
- ◆ Do 35 sit-ups. Try 35 straight—no rest.
- ◆ Do 15 lunges on the walk. No rest in between lunges.
- ◆ Walk 40 minutes—include 5 intervals. You decide on the intensity and duration.
- ◆ Stretch.

Schedule your appointments now:

Monday

Friday

Tuesday

Saturday

Wednesday

Sunday

Thursday

* SPECIAL *
ASSIGNMENT

- ◆ Draw up a weekly time budget.
- ◆ Take a casual evening stroll every
  night this week after dinner.

_T_o_e RAISE

Yahoo! This is the start of our sixth and final month. So far, we've covered five of your body's major muscle groups: the heart with walking; abdominals with sit-ups; triceps and pectorals with push-ups; quadriceps, hamstrings, and gluteals with the lunge; and biceps and forearms with curls. Now we're going to concentrate on the calf by adding toe raises.

The toe raise is an excellent exercise that tones the calves, strengthens the ankles, and increases your endurance while on your feet. It's a great stretch for the achilles and can help prevent ankle injuries.

In fact, this simple exercise should be mandatory for those who wear high heels. Ladies, be sure to do your Betty Grables!

Now, let's try a toe raise. I've found the best way to do toe raises is on a stairstep or curb. They can be done on a flat surface, but this limits the range of motion.

Okay, find something to hold onto for balance. Stand on the balls of your feet with your heels hanging off the stair so that your calf muscles (gastrocs) are fully stretched. Next, contract your calves by bringing your heels as high above the stair as possible. Slowly lower your heels back to the original position and you've done a complete toe raise. Be sure to do the exercise slowly; don't bounce and remember to breathe.

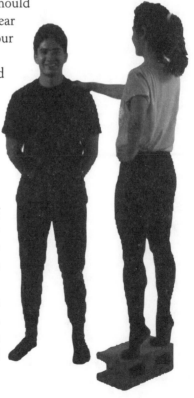

TRIVIA

If you get a muscle cramp
in your leg, try pinching the
middle of your top lip.
Ahhh, relief!!

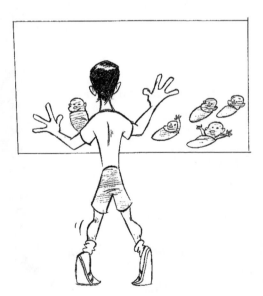

Toe raises can be done anywhere.

Duffy Fitness

Hi, I tried to reach you but your line was busy. I had to dash out of town 'cuz my sister's having a baby!

While I'm gone, I want you to design your own program. Write down the three appointments and be sure to include one challenge. Add in a couple of special assignments from the past, like self-massage or a catnap. I know you can do it, so, good luck. I'll see you next week.

Uncle Duf

Duf

P.S. Don't forget to add toe raises. Try 10 for starters.

☐ **Appointment #1**

- ◆ Do 10 toe raises.
- ◆ Do ___ curls.
- ◆ Do ___ push-ups.
- ◆ Do ___ sit-ups.
- ◆ Do ___ lunges during the walk.
- ◆ Walk ___ minutes.
- ◆ Stretch.

☐ **Appointment #2**

- ◆ Do ___ toe raises.
- ◆ Do ___ curls.
- ◆ Do ___ push-ups.
- ◆ Do ___ sit-ups.
- ◆ Do ___ lunges during the walk.
- ◆ Walk ___ minutes. CHALLENGE: ___ intervals of __ seconds each.
- ◆ Stretch.

☐ **Appointment #3**

- ◆ Do ___ toe raises.
- ◆ Do ___ curls.
- ◆ Do ___ push-ups.
- ◆ Do ___ sit-ups.
- ◆ Do ___ lunges during the walk.
- ◆ Take your RHR, write it down on your Vital Statistics chart. Any change?
- ◆ Walk ___ minutes.
- ◆ Stretch.

Schedule your appointments now:

Monday

Friday

Tuesday

Saturday

Wednesday

Sunday

Thursday

* SPECIAL *
ASSIGNMENT

You choose: _____

_____

_____

_____

_____

TRIVIA

Exercise and Eat Accordingly

Your metabolism is the sum of the energy used by all the cells of your body. We've all seen people who eat constantly and don't gain an ounce. It doesn't mean they're healthy, but it probably means they have a high metabolism. Make the distinction between healthy and fortunate. Your metabolic rate increases during exercise and remains elevated for a couple of hours afterward. Understand your body's metabolism.

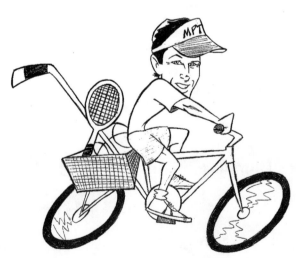

Add a little spice to your good health program.

Hi. It's a girl! Believe it or not, my sister had a 10-pounder. Wow! Uncle Duf is stoked.

Well, how did the appointments go last week? Since we only have 3 more weeks together, last week was a perfect time to prepare yourself to keep exercising on your own. I hope you will join my former clients who continue to practice good health.

This week, let's add a little spice to your program.

When's the last time you played tennis, shot baskets, swam, or rode a bike? Check out the Alternative Exercise section (pg. 141) and come back. Pick an activity right now and write it down as a fourth appointment. I want you to promise to try it, even if it's only for 10 minutes.

In the future, you may enjoy supplementing your routine with a sport you haven't played in years or a brand new activity. Try it on a rest day. It's a nice way to stay involved with others and to keep moving.

I'm going ice skating,

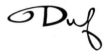

P.S. How did your toe raises go last week? For an added challenge, hold the up position for 10 seconds. Don't forget to breathe!

☐ **Appointment #1**

- ◆ Do 15 toe raises.
- ◆ Do 15 curls—do all the exercises slowly. Focus on your form.
- ◆ Do 15 push-ups.
- ◆ Do 35 sit-ups.
- ◆ Do 15 lunges.
- ◆ Walk 35 minutes—take it easy today.
- ◆ Stretch.

☐ **Appointment #2**

- ◆ Do ___ toe raises.
- ◆ Do ___ curls.
- ◆ Do ___ push-ups.
- ◆ Do ___ sit-ups.
- ◆ Do ___ lunges.
- ◆ Walk 30 minutes. CHALLENGE—increase the distance of your walk. The "Breathing" section (pg. 122) will give you some helpful hints for recovery.
- ◆ Stretch.

☐ **Appointment #3**

- ◆ Do 15 toe raises.
- ◆ Do 15 curls.
- ◆ Do 15 push-ups.
- ◆ Do 40 sit-ups.
- ◆ Do 15 lunges.
- ◆ Walk 40 minutes. Take an easy walk and include eight 10-second intervals.
- ◆ Stretch.

☐ **Appointment #4**

- ◆ Select an alternative activity: _____.

Schedule your appointments now:

Monday	Friday
Tuesday	**Saturday**
Wednesday	**Sunday**
Thursday	

★ SPECIAL ★
ASSIGNMENT

"The foot bone's connected to the ankle bone." Of the body's 206 bones, 52 are in the feet. A good foot exercise is to draw the letters of the alphabet in the air with your toes. Do it now and follow with a quick foot massage.

TRIVIA

Time for Duf's *Airobics*

Jet lag can be reduced
tremendously with exercise
and a good frame of mind.
When boarding, set your
watch and your mind to
your destination's time. In
flight, drink plenty of H_2O
and move about often.
Upon arrival, take a walk to
get the blood flowing.
You'll sleep easier and wake
up refreshed.

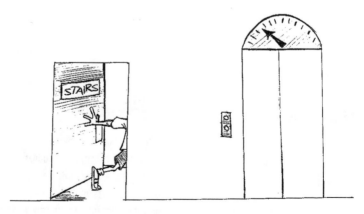

Exercise is a mind-set. Expect to move.

Sweet! Only 2 more weeks until you're on your own. By the way, how did the new activity go last week? Try it again soon—a little diversity can enhance your existing program and help keep you moving.

Since exercise is now a fundamental part of your life, here are a few tips to keep you going. First, establish *realistic goals*. Remember when we met? We had a 6-month goal during which you would practice good health and I would help you learn a basic exercise regime.

A future goal might be to go for another 6 months. No, you don't have to buy a second copy of *My Personal Trainer* (darn!) because I've provided blank appointment pages (pg. 144), which you can copy and use to design your own program. Or, how about training for a 10K walk? Get a friend to join you and check out a walking magazine for a training program. Maybe you want to try tennis lessons or join a hiking club. See your local YMCA.

Remember, *exercise is a mind-set*. If you expect to move, soon you'll find yourself doing interesting things like taking the stairs instead of the elevator, parking a little farther from the office, or going on a family walk while the Thanksgiving turkey is roasting.

Speaking of holidays, if you travel (business or pleasure), exercise is a great way to combat jet lag or a long car ride. Bring your walking shoes and weather-appropriate attire so you can maintain your program. The point is, *keep moving.*

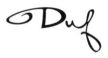

☐ **Appointment #1**

- ◆ Do ___ toe raises.
- ◆ Do ___ curls.
- ◆ Do ___ push-ups.
- ◆ Do ___ sit-ups.
- ◆ Do ___ lunges.
- ◆ Walk 45 minutes—grab a tennis ball for your forearms.
- ◆ Stretch.

☐ **Appointment #2**

- ◆ Today, do the exercises slowly and concentrate on your form.
- ◆ Do 10 toe raises.
- ◆ Do 10 curls.
- ◆ Do 10 push-ups.
- ◆ Do 20 sit-ups.
- ◆ Do 10 lunges.
- ◆ Walk 45 minutes.
- ◆ Stretch.

☐ **Appointment #3**

- ◆ Do 10 toe raises.
- ◆ Do 10 curls.
- ◆ Do 10 push-ups.
- ◆ Do 20 sit-ups.
- ◆ Do 10 lunges.
- ◆ Walk 45 minutes.
- ◆ Stretch.

Schedule your appointments now:

Monday	**Friday**
Tuesday	**Saturday**
Wednesday	**Sunday**
Thursday	

* SPECIAL *
ASSIGNMENT

When you go out this week, park your car a few blocks from your destination. It's an easy way to get a little extra movement.

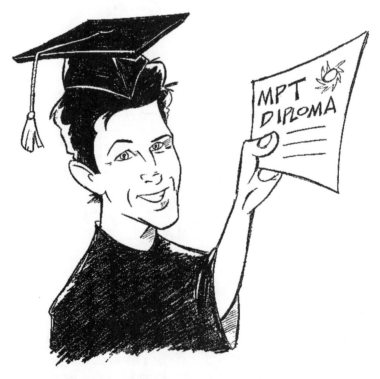

Congratulations. Keep practicing good health.

Congratulations! Over the past 6 months you've acquired the tools to continue exercising on your own. Even if you only did the walking part of this program, you've taken steps in the right direction to improve your health. Hopefully, I've been a good "coach" and you've learned a lot about yourself. You're fortunate to have a functioning body. Use it and take special care of it.

Remember, to err is human. We all will skip exercise or eat the wrong foods. *Moderation and practice* will help you stay on track. Refer to me as needed to help remind you to listen to your body and practice good health.

Be proud of who you are. Although you can't change genetics, you do control the three most important aspects of a healthy lifestyle: *exercise, diet,* and *rest.*

Finally, I want you to use the following measure as your fitness "gold standard":

Walk for 30 minutes.

The rest is up to you. Mix it up and have fun!

I'm very proud of you. I hope our paths cross again, until then,

Practice good health!

Your Personal Trainer,

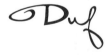

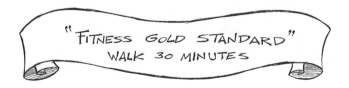

"Fitness Gold Standard"
Walk 30 Minutes

☐ Appointment #1

- ◆ Do 15 toe raises.
- ◆ Do 15 curls.
- ◆ Do 15 push-ups.
- ◆ Do 40 sit-ups.
- ◆ Do 15 lunges.
- ◆ Walk 40 minutes.
- ◆ Stretch.

☐ Appointment #2

- ◆ Do 15 toe raises.
- ◆ Do 15 curls.
- ◆ Do 15 push-ups.
- ◆ Do 40 sit-ups.
- ◆ Do 15 lunges.
- ◆ Walk 40 minutes.
- ◆ Stretch.

☐ Appointment #3

- ◆ Do 20 toe raises.
- ◆ Do 20 curls.
- ◆ Do 20 push-ups.
- ◆ Do 40 sit-ups.
- ◆ Do 20 lunges.
- ◆ Walk 45 minutes—try one 10-second interval every minute for 10 consecutive minutes. I know; it's tough!
- ◆ Stretch.
- ◆ There's no better way to end the week than by giving yourself a full body massage. Keep up the good work!

Schedule your appointments now:

Monday

Friday

Tuesday

Saturday

Wednesday

Sunday

Thursday

* SPECIAL *
ASSIGNMENT

Give up a bad habit this week. Write
it down: _____

_____.

Abstain as long as you can. Use the
money or time you save to treat
yourself. You deserve it.

CHAPTER EIGHT
GOOD HEALTH READINGS

Vital Statistics

NAME: _____   **HEIGHT:** _____

AGE: _____   **WEIGHT:** _____

Resting Heart Rate (RHR)	
Mo1-Wk1	
Mo2-Wk1	
Mo3-Wk1	
Mo4-Wk1	
Mo5-Wk1	
Mo6-Wk1	

Maximum Heart Rate (MAX HR) : _____

Target Heart Rate (THR) : _____to_____
                               (60% MAX HR)   (90% MAX HR)

Body Type

Ectomorph (Thin) _____
Endomorph (Thick) _____
Mesomorph (Muscular) _____

Goals

Tone _____
Strength _____
Weight Gain-Loss _____

Blood Volume : _____

The S.A.I.D. Principle:
Use It Or Lose It

Now that you've made the commitment to exercise, aren't you curious as to how it will change your body over the next 6 months?

Let me introduce you to the S.A.I.D. principle: *Specific Adaptations to Imposed Demands*. Simply stated, your body changes (adapts) to the stresses (in this case, exercises) placed upon it. Think about it.

Did Magic Johnson learn how to play basketball by practicing tennis? Of course not. The body responds to the tasks put upon it.

For example, later in the program I introduce the push-up. At first, it may be a struggle to do only 1 or 2. That's okay. When you do a couple of them, a new demand is placed on the muscles of your arms and back. The muscle fibers in these areas break down and rebuild stronger to be ready for this new demand. In time, 2 push-ups are a piece of cake; your muscles have adapted. Now, you'll be attempting 5 push-ups. Once again, your muscle fibers break down and rebuild even stronger.

As you can see, the S.A.I.D. principle is rather simple: your body adapts to what you ask of it. If you want to run faster, practice running fast. If you want to lift a car over your head, forget it! Obviously, there is a physiological limit.

Since our objective is overall health, I've designed this program with the S.A.I.D. principle in mind. Walking imposes demands on your whole body, especially your heart. And the five additional exercises that are added to the program, such as the push-up, strengthen each major muscle group.

By the way, if you don't move your body, guess what? That's right, the use it or lose it theory also applies.

So, remember the S.A.I.D. principle, I'll be referring to it often. Now, if you want to start feeling good, you need to do one more thing: take the first step... and let your body respond.

The Matter of the Heart

Make a fist. Did you know that's the approximate size of your heart? Pretty amazing, huh? This relatively small muscle beats about 100,000 times to pump blood on a 168,000-mile journey through your arteries and veins. Every day! How would you like that job? Well, you don't have to consciously do the work, but you are the boss. So, your job is to protect and care for your heart—the most important muscle you have.

The heart delivers nourishment and oxygen to all 45 trillion cells in your body. If your heart doesn't work right, you don't work right. I like to think of the heart as the body's battery, and cardiovascular exercise, such as walking, keeps it charged.

Remember the S.A.I.D. (Specific Adaptations to Imposed Demands) principle introduced earlier? The more you exercise, the more you ask of your heart, which responds by getting bigger, stronger, and more efficient. Since walking is the foundation of this program, your heart will get the exercise it needs to give you the stamina you need.

Resting Heart Rate (RHR):
Month One–Week One

Now, let's pause for a moment and observe your heart in action. Before you open your eyes in the morning, your heart is relaxed and beating the minimum number of times to keep you alive. This is your heart's slowest pace, also known as Resting Heart Rate (RHR).

The alarm rings. You roll over, punch it off, and sit up. Now, more muscles are moving and your heart beats faster. Then, you get out of bed and head to the kitchen. Each added activity causes your heart to beat fast enough for you to perform the task(s). You get the picture. The more you move the more you ask your heart to work. With a weak heart, even the simple task of getting out of bed can be stressful; and a big task like shoveling snow can be fatal.

We're going to check your RHR once a month throughout this program. This will help you monitor your heart's efficiency. As your health improves and your heart gets stronger, your RHR should decrease. When the heart is strong, it pumps blood at a slower pace (i.e., fewer beats). For instance, world class marathon runners have RHR's in the low 30's. Ours will be considerably higher, falling within the range of 60 to 90 beats per minute.

Okay, let's calculate your RHR.

The best way is to take your RHR in the morning while in bed before you move a muscle.

(1) Locate your pulse by grasping your right hand around your left wrist (palms facing you).

(2) Count the number of beats for 60 seconds (use a clock).

(3) Write down your RHR on your Vital Statistics chart (pg. 117).

(4) When taking your RHR, be consistent. Always take the measurement at the same time of day, preferably first thing in the morning before you get out of bed.

Maximum Heart Rate (MAX HR):
Month One–Week Two

Now, let's look at Maximum Heart Rate (MAX HR). This measurement means just that—the maximum number of times your heart can beat in 1 minute. You can find your MAX HR through a simple formula:

$$220 - \text{your age} = \text{your MAX HR.}$$

Obviously, everyone your age doesn't have the exact same heart or the same MAX HR, so add or subtract 10 beats per minute. Your MAX HR will fall into that zone. For example, if you are 40 years old, your MAX HR is in the range of 170 to 190 (220 - 40 = 180 +/- 10). If you are 30 years old, your MAX HR falls between 180 and 200. It's an interesting personal statistic. Write your MAX HR on your Vitals because we'll need it next week.

Target Heart Rate (THR):
Month One–Week Three

Anyone who exercises will eventually come across the term Target Heart Rate (THR). THR is a measurement used to indicate that you have elevated your heart rate enough to benefit from exercise. THR can be used as a goal during intense exercise such as the walking intervals. However, I find it cumbersome and often confusing.

I believe you benefit from walking the moment you step foot out the door. Furthermore, hard breathing during the intervals is a good indicator that you are challenging yourself. It is often awkward to stop and take your pulse and check a watch to determine if you're within the THR.

Still, as your personal trainer, it is my professional obligation to keep you abreast of fashionable exercise lingo.

To calculate your THR, take 60 percent and 90 percent of your maximum heart rate. This is your THR zone. After you complete a walking interval or similar challenge, take a moment to find your pulse. Count the beats for 10 seconds and multiply that number by 6. That's your current heart rate (HR). If it falls between 60 and 90 percent of your MAX HR, then you have reached your target.

Let's say you are 20 years old; your MAX HR is 220 - your age +/- 10. So, your MAX HR is 190 to 210. If you multiply that by 60 to 90 percent, your THR is 114 to 189 beats per minute or 19 to 31 beats per 10 seconds. Go ahead and calculate your THR now. Write it on the Vitals chart.

As you can see, this is a fairly broad range. Keep in mind, I will ask you to challenge yourself at times during our walks. If monitoring your heart rate to see if you're in your THR zone helps you, fine. However, if the calculations slow you down, then don't bother. I prefer you keep moving and listen to your body by using your breathing rate to indicate how hard you are exercising.

Breathing

The breathing reflex is involuntary. And it's a good thing, too, because we breathe about 22,000 times a day. If it weren't automatic, none of us would get anything done! Imagine, "hold on a second, I'm trying to remember to breathe."

Breathing is an exchange of two gases between the body and the environment. The first, oxygen (O_2), provides fuel for your tissues. The second, carbon dioxide (CO_2), is the exhaust.

There's an interesting misconception about breathing—that we breathe to take in oxygen (O_2). Actually, the breathing reflex is triggered to eliminate carbon dioxide (CO_2).

Oxygen intake occurs freely once the breathing muscles (diaphragm) have relaxed. Try it... exhale fully, now relax and feel your lungs fill with air. Once your lungs are full, if you remain relaxed, nothing happens. To get another breath, you need to contract your diaphragm muscle. It is exhaling, not inhaling, that keeps you breathing.

When walking at a casual pace, you may not even be aware of your breathing patterns. However, during a challenge such as the interval walks, your breaths will become shorter and quicker. If you're not accustomed to being winded, you may feel like you'll never catch your breath again. Try not to panic, because this will make your breaths even more rapid.

Here's the best way I've found to catch my breath, known as *recovery breathing*.

(1) Keep moving at an easy pace. This is important because the muscles will continue to contract, which helps move the blood back to the heart and lungs.

(2) Put both hands on top of your head. This opens the chest cavity, which allows the lungs more room for expansion.

(3) Breathe consciously. Begin by taking a deep breath and holding it for 2 or 3 seconds. Do it again and, if necessary, once more.

(4) Then, move on to taking slow, deep breaths. Inhale and exhale fully. This will enable you to find a relaxed breathing rhythm during the walk.

Practice this method and soon you'll be able to control your breathing during strenuous walking.

The good news is as you become more fit, your recovery period (the time it takes breathing to normalize) will shorten. How, you ask? Picture your lungs and circulatory system as a highway where little trucks transport O_2 and CO_2. Over time, your body adapts to the demands of walking by manufacturing more trucks to deliver the gases more efficiently. Walking and breathing seem easier. They *are* easier. The S.A.I.D. (Specific Adaptations to Imposed Demands) principle strikes again.

P.S. Controlled breathing is a great tool when experiencing stress, anger, or fear. Remain calm, close your mouth, and slowly inhale and exhale fully through your nose. Try this a couple of times. It will give you time to collect your thoughts before acting out.

Stretching

Stretching is vital to any exercise program. Exercise contracts and shortens the muscles; stretching lengthens and relaxes them. Additionally, stretching provides an important opportunity to develop body awareness by identifying tight muscles.

When you stretch, avoid bouncing or jerking. Forget the old phys-ed coach's commands. Ballistic stretching can shred your muscle fibers. That's why we do *static stretching.* For this method, we stretch the muscle slowly as far as possible and then hold that position. As you hold, the muscle begins to relax, lengthening further, and the stretch can be extended. Repeat this procedure until you feel an adequate stretch, then move on to the next muscle. *Here are some guidelines.*

I want you to stretch twice during each appointment:

First, a few minutes into the walk, after the muscles have warmed up, do each of the 10 stretches briefly (about 10 seconds each). Perhaps you've noticed athletes loosening up before competition. A slightly stretched muscle is at its optimum length, which not only leads to better performance, but prevents injury.

Secondly, after our appointment, take time to do all 10 stretches leisurely. I usually spend between 30 seconds and 3 minutes on each stretch. This is a time to relax the muscle groups and to identify tight areas. *Listen to your body* and spend some extra time stretching when needed. Take a few deep breaths and rub the muscles to help them relax. Over time, your flexibility will improve and your body will love you for it.

Heeerrre Are the 10 Stretches

There are zillions of stretches. I've chosen 10 that cover all the major muscle groups. Each stretch can be done from a standing position. Keep your feet shoulder-width apart with toes pointed forward, unless otherwise instructed. Stretching can seem difficult at first, so take your time and keep practicing. Eventually, you may find yourself stretching even when you're not exercising. Go for it, it's a great way to keep the blood flowing.

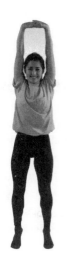

1. Morning Stretch.

Interlock your fingers on both hands and raise your arms high above your head. Get them up a little higher by standing on your tiptoes. This is easy and will wake you up.

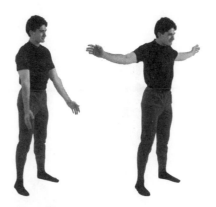

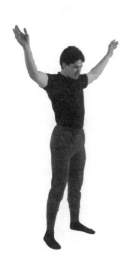

2. Big Circles.

With your arms extended, simultaneously rotate both arms all the way around in big circles 5 times. Then reverse directions for 5 more. This gets the blood pumping and loosens up your shoulders.

3. Trunk Rotation.

Interlock fingers with arms raised in front of you at shoulder level. Rotate trunk from side to side 3 times each way. Be sure to do each rotation slowly and hold it for a few seconds when you've gone as far as you can. You should feel this stretch mainly in your upper back and shoulders.

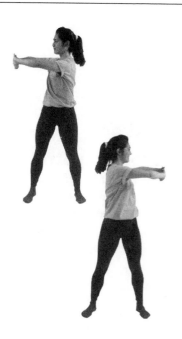

4. Hang Down.

Slowly bend over at the waist and walk your hands down their respective legs. The goal is to touch your toes with only a slight bend at the knees. You should feel this in the backs of your legs (hamstrings).

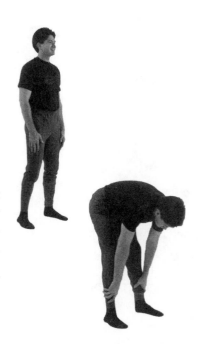

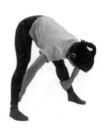

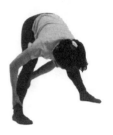

5. Pull Thru.

Still hanging from the "hang down" position, spread your legs a little wider. (Remember to keep your feet pointing forward.) Grab the inside of each leg with its respective arm and try to pull your upper body between your legs. It won't happen, but you'll feel a little better stretch on the backs of your legs and lower back. Now, while in the same position, take both arms over to one leg and try to touch your head to your knee. Switch legs. Remember, the stretch is the important thing. Don't be discouraged if you can't touch your head to your knee. I can rarely do it.

6. Groin Stretch.

With your feet still wider than shoulder-width, your toes still pointing forward, and your upper body facing ahead, keep one leg straight and bend the other leg into a squatting position. You should feel this stretch on the inner thigh of your straight leg. One important point: to get the most out of this stretch, keep both feet flat on the ground pointing forward. If it helps, widen your stance.

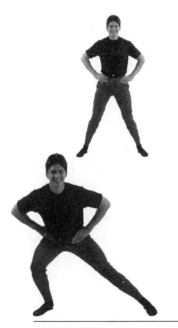

7. Quad Stretch.

For this stretch, find a stable support such as a wall or handrail to lean against. Stand upright and put one arm against the support for balance, grab your ankle with your free hand, and pull so that you feel a stretch on the front part of your leg (quadriceps). Switch legs.

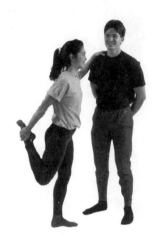

8. Calf Stretch.

Using the same support as for the quad stretch, lean against it with one leg straight and your body at an angle. Be sure to find the angle where your heel is barely off the ground so you feel your calf stretching. Switch legs.

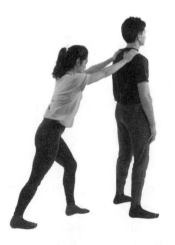

9. Side Stretch.

Stand with feet slightly wider than shoulder-width and toes pointing forward. With both hands on your hips, lean slowly to the left, then the right. Make sure you lean to the side and not forward or backward. As you get better at this stretch, you can take one hand away from your hip and reach over your head as you lean to the side. You should feel this stretch all along your trunk.

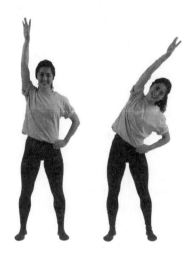

10. Head Roll.

Put your chin to your chest and roll your head clockwise, then counterclockwise. Then, looking straight ahead without moving your shoulders, turn your head as far to the left and then as far to the right as possible. Go slowly, so you feel your neck muscles stretch.

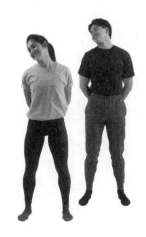

Duf's Cantina—Menu Du Jour

Upon arising:

I like to start the day with a glass of water to hydrate my body. I don't eat until I've been up and moving around for about 1 hour (for example, after a shower and shave).

Breakfast:

Think of breakfast as a snack. Unless you're a lumberjack, the BIG BREAKFAST is a big myth. Listen to your body. A light breakfast that is easily digested is best.

Midmorning snack:

Your midmorning snack may be a little more or a little less than breakfast. I listen to my body and eat just enough to carry me over until lunch.

Lunch:

Usually, lunch is my biggest meal of the day. I don't pig out, but I do believe this is the time of day when the body can best handle a little more volume. I prefer not to read or work over lunch, so I can enjoy the eating experience.

Midafternoon snack:

A midafternoon snack is optional, depending on my dinner plans and on what my body is saying.

Dinner:

Dinner is usually smaller than lunch. When eating out, I've been known to order only salad and an appetizer. If you feel obligated to clear your plate (yes, many in the world are starving), then take smaller portions. Here are a couple tips: Share dessert—everyone gets a taste! Finish dinner no later than 2 hours before bedtime. You want your body to sleep at night, not digest.

Late-night snack:

Keep late-night snacks light. Better yet, drink a glass of water! This can keep the munchies at bay.

The above isn't carved in stone; it's just some food for thought. Listen to your body.

Shopping for Nutrition

Our first good health practice is to exercise regularly; the second is to eat healthfully. Eating well can be an easy and pleasurable experience. All it takes is a little planning, some guidance from the Food Pyramid, and a trip to a good local market. Oh yes, don't forget a pre-shopping snack—it's dangerous to hit the market hungry. I've known times where a bag of chips disappeared between aisles 10 and 12!

Take a careful look at the Food Pyramid below. Better yet, tear it out and tape it on the fridge for future reference. The Pyramid will help you figure out how much of each food group to buy. Keep in mind that most healthful foods are fresh, unprocessed, and without preservatives. So, plan to shop accordingly, perhaps every few days. Be honest when drawing up a grocery list and stick to it once you're in the store. This will make it easier not to grab the cookies off the shelf. (What cookies? They're not on the list!)

Okay. With all this in mind, grab a cart and let's go!

Food Guide Pyramid

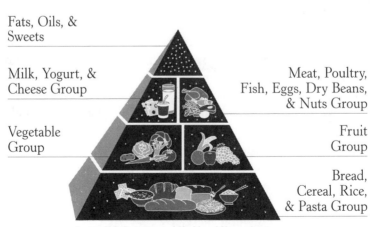

Fats, Oils, & Sweets

Milk, Yogurt, & Cheese Group

Meat, Poultry, Fish, Eggs, Dry Beans, & Nuts Group

Vegetable Group

Fruit Group

Bread, Cereal, Rice, & Pasta Group

Source: U.S. Department of Health and Human Services

Duf's Grocery List

Fruits/Vegetables

Produce is the foundation of my diet. Fresh fruits and vegetables are excellent sources of vitamins, minerals, and complex carbohydrates. They also provide necessary fiber to keep the digestive tract working properly.

Choose produce carefully. Make sure it is fresh, ripe, and in good condition. If locally grown or organic, all the better.

Pick an array of colors. This is an easy way to make sure your body receives the various vitamins and minerals it needs. I eat a salad a day, but if you're not into salads, how about lettuce, tomato, and onion on your next sandwich?

Fruits are great for breakfast or snacks. I like fruit juice on my cereal, and I keep a piece of fruit in my car for a quick munchy.

Don't overlook fresh herbs, garlic, lemons, and limes. These items can add zest and flavor to steamed veggies, salads, and fresh fruit. They are healthful alternatives to butter, salt, and pepper.

Bread/Cereal/Rice/Pasta

These items are also important sources of carbohydrates and fiber.

I try to buy these foods in their natural state (for example, brown rice, whole grain cereals, and sprouted wheat breads). My favorites from this group are whole grain cereal and freshly baked multi-grained bread.

Get out your spectacles and read food labels. This can be a real eye opener, let alone a tongue twister. Keep away from additives, preservatives, and processed ingredients.

Meat/Poultry/Fish/Dry Beans/Eggs/Nuts

These are the primary sources of protein. It's okay to eat red meat occasionally, but remember, no matter how lean, it still contains a high amount of fat and cholesterol. Fish and skinless poultry are healthful meat alternatives.

Your body needs only about 6 ounces of protein each day. Most unused protein is converted and stored as fat. It's helpful to remember that 4 ounces of meat is about the size of a deck of cards and ½ cup is about one handful.

I am especially careful when I shop for meats. I usually buy free range chicken and meats that are free of hormones and antibodies. They cost more, but I only need small portions.

I like to eat two or three eggs a week. How about a hardboiled egg as a convenient snack?

Dry beans are perfect for soup; a meal that will last a few days.

Raw, unsalted nuts are excellent sprinkled on salads and handy for quick snacks.

Milk/Yogurt/Cheese

These are good sources of calcium and protein. If you want to lose weight (fat), choose low-fat products from this group.

Try low-fat milk on your whole grain cereal with fresh fruit added. How about nonfat yogurt? Be sure to check the label for additives and sweeteners.

Hard cheeses (cheddar, Parmesan, Romano) have less fat. Goat cheese is often easier to digest. If you really miss butter, then use less of the real thing. Margarines and other fake butters are processed.

Other Items

Caffeinated drinks (coffee, tea, and sodas) and junk foods (cookies, chips, and candy) are not nutritious. Worse yet, caffeine dehydrates you and causes the depletion of nutrients already absorbed into your body. Junk foods are on the tip of the Food Pyramid— the smallest section. You flat out don't need these calories. If you crave a snack, how about an apple with cheese?

Shopping for nutrition can be ridiculously simple. A nurse friend of mine tells her patients to *shop the perimeter* of grocery stores. That's just what we've done. Check your list before venturing into the other aisles, read labels, and be selective. Remember, the three most important aspects of the foods you choose are quality, quality, quality.

Let's Go Shopping
Grocery List

_____   _____

_____   _____

_____   _____

_____   _____

_____   _____

_____   _____

_____   _____

_____   _____

_____   _____

_____   _____

_____   _____

_____   _____

_____   _____

Throw-Away-Your-Diet-Book Diet

...And while you're at it, get rid of the bathroom scale. From this point on, I want you to rely on the mirror. Why? First of all, a handful of muscles weighs 10 times more than a handful of fat. Also, 60 percent of your body weight is water. So, if you put on some muscle, lose a bunch of fat, and drink a couple glasses of water, what's the scale going to tell you? *Your weight is not necessarily a measure of your health.*

However, if your mirror suggests that you are overweight, and you want to shed some pounds, then you've come to the right place.

Weight Loss U.—Where U Lose Weight.
Mission Statement

Founded on the simple principle that weight loss is accomplished by eating healthy foods and exercising more, WLU offers a full curriculum. It is our philosophy that over time the body slowly adapts to extra pounds. Our motto: "You didn't gain weight overnight, you're not going to lose it overnight."

Admissions

All applicants are accepted since this is a home-based program. The courses are not bound by time constraint. However, a reasonable weight loss schedule is 1 pound per week.

Course Catalog

Genetics 101: Required. In-depth examination reveals that we can't all be Arnold Schwarzenegger or Raquel Welch. Students identify and learn to accept their own God-given body type:

♦ *Endomorph*—the soft, round form with larger arms and thighs, sometimes referred to as "plump."

♦ *Ectomorph*—the linear physique with somewhat delicate bone structure, often referred to as "skinny."

♦ *Mesomorph*—a somewhat rectangular physique featuring heavy, hard muscles; "muscular."

Advanced Genome Theory: Laboratory. DNA manipulation to alter body type: not offered during your lifetime. *Accept your own morph.*

21st Century Realism: A short course to determine a sensible weight loss goal based on the theorem: "calories consumed (food eaten) minus calories burned (exercise) = pounds gained or lost." An expected and safe schedule is to *lose 1 pound per week.*

I'm Okay, You're Okay: Introductory self-help course whereby students learn basic politically correct thinking. For example, "good and bad" foods are redefined as "healthful" and "unhealthful." Don't feel guilty if you eat a pint of ice cream. *Practice, practice, practice good health habits.* It takes time to change.

Metabolic Rate Analysis: (Mandatory). An in-depth examination of the physiology of weight loss based on the complex chemical and physical relationship between calories burned and calories consumed.

Are you kidding? Whaddya think this is, Med School? Simply put: prolonged aerobic exercise, such as walking, burns calories. This caloric consumption continues for a few hours following exercise. Thus, if you wish to lose weight, follow the walking program and refrain from eating for a couple of hours after exercise.

Facilities

Your home and neighborhood. Students are advised to avoid common cafeteria offerings, such as coffee, sodas, cookies, and chips.

Bottom line...

There are no secret formulas for losing weight. Be wary of quick weight loss schemes. They don't work! The only way to control weight is through consistent exercise and a healthful diet.

Spot Reducing

Surely you've heard of a brand new special kind of sit-up that will melt the fat from your stomach. Or, a one-of-a-kind machine guaranteed to trim inches off your thighs. Well, guess what? Phooey! *You cannot spot reduce.*

Spot reducing is a gimmick used to sell products. Don't be fooled. It's true, certain exercises can tone isolated muscles, but you can't select a specific area to burn fat.

That said, let's chew some fat....

The good news about fat is that it is a necessary and critical body component. It insulates and protects your vital organs, such as your heart, liver, and kidneys. And if you could see inside yourself, you'd find fat located around your muscles, nerves, and brain.

The visible fat on your body is protection against extended periods without food. Remember, not too long ago there were no such thing as grocery stores. It was not unusual to go one or two days without eating, and the stored fat became an emergency energy source.

Perhaps you've noticed men and women store fat differently. Men tend to store fat in the stomach area, better known as a pot belly. Women, on the other hand, have babies, and since fat doesn't stretch, the stomach isn't a good spot to store excess fat. Thus, nature provided women with storage compartments in their thighs and backs of the arms.

You are born with the total number of fat cells that remain with you throughout life. Think of these fat cells as empty storage containers that shrink or swell depending on food consumed and energy burned. The theory is that once you have a fat cell, you cannot lose it; you can only fill or empty it. The only true (healthy) way to eliminate fat from the storage container is to burn more energy than you consume.

If all your fat cells are filled and you continue to consume fat, the existing fat cells may divide thus increasing your storage capacity.

The body chooses which fat cells it will empty for needed fuel. Don't be surprised if your face thins before your thighs. You cannot spot reduce!

No matter where your trouble spots are located, the best way to lose fat is through cardiovascular exercise, like walking.

Now, let's burn some fat.

Rest

Kicking up your feet, sawing logs, or catching some Z's, rest comes in many different forms. No matter how you do it, you need to rest about 8 hours a day.

Rest, our third good health practice is a quiet time of ease when we relax and refresh ourselves.

Sleeping, the most important form of rest, rejuvenates the brain. Surprisingly, your body can function without rest but your brain can't. In fact, sleep deprivation causes the brain to malfunction, which can lead to abnormal activities.

I recommend establishing a fairly consistent sleep routine. Try to eat at least 2 hours before you go to bed. This enables the body to rest during sleep instead of doing the work of digesting dinner.

Open a window for fresh air and turn down the heat—if necessary, add an extra blanket. Finally, be sure to turn off the television to give yourself some quiet time before looking at the back of your eyelids. On the days you are suffering from lack of sleep, that mid-day coffee or soda is not the "refresh"ment your mind needs.

A better way to recharge is to take a *10-minute catnap.* You may have hated 'em in kindergarten, but you'll love them as an adult.

Catnaps are simple. The objective is to be able to close your eyes for exactly 10 minutes. Lying down is best, but sitting back in a chair or putting your head on the desk will do. Shut your eyes, and if you open them before the 10 minutes are up, shut them again. With some practice, your body will develop an internal alarm. Who knows, perhaps you'll even dream!

Natural rest is a vital element of healthful living. Drug-induced sleep via pills or alcohol robs the body of important time it has to take care of itself.

Listen to your body and remember the catnap if fatigued. The 10 minutes will give you the needed energy boost to keep going. Polish your napping skills. Give the catnap a try right now. Z-Z-Z-Z-Z.

Self-Massage

Ever had a full-body massage? Well, even if you haven't, it's time to try one. A professional masseur will charge some dough; and yes, it's worth it. However, you won't need any cash for this experience.

Self-massage is one of the most relaxing things you can do. It enables you to get in "touch" with your body from the tip of your littlest toe to the hair on your head.

Self-massage stimulates areas that rarely get attention. When did you last spend a minute rubbing your ears? How about your eyeballs or the bottoms of your feet? Massaging these areas is easy, yet most of us never think of doing it.

Self-massage helps stimulate blood flow, relieves muscle soreness, and is magnificent for *developing body awareness*. Plus, it feels great!

A Self-Massage Primer

Here's where: Find a comfortable, quiet spot where you won't be disturbed (i.e., bedroom). Turn on some easy tunes if you desire, sit down, and go for it.

Attire: Stark naked or shorts only is the best. Remember, it's your body, so don't be shy.

Here's how: Start with the feet and work your way up. One at a time, grab your toes, twist your ankles, stroke the bottoms of your feet—whatever tickles your fancy.

After each foot, massage each leg. Be thorough. For example, rub the muscles, tendons, and bony areas. Utilize long strokes, deep pressure, soft pressure, or any movement that is pleasurable. Everyone is different, so decide what your body likes. You can't go wrong.

After you finish the lower extremities, lie down and massage the stomach area. Continue with the trunk, sides, chest, and arms.

Then move on to my favorite areas: the head and neck. Get your neck, chin, cheeks, lips, nose, ears, eyes, forehead, and scalp.

I give myself a full-body massage at least once a month, for 20 minutes to 1 hour each session. Plus, I perform a brief localized rubdown on my face, knees, or feet almost every day. Remember, it's your body. Give self-massage a try, and with some practice, you'll figure out what feels good.

Alternative Exercises and Various Activities

Exercises:

Jogging–Works the cardiovascular system.

Stationary bike–Works the cardiovascular system.

Rowing machine–Works the cardiovascular system. It also helps improve your upper body strength. (Be careful of your back!)

Weight lifting–Strengthens muscles, depending on type of exercises used.

Jump rope–Works cardiovascular system, also causes some gains in both upper and lower body strength.

Aerobics–Works cardiovascular system, also strengthens and tones muscles.

Yoga–Excellent way to work on flexibility and breathing techniques.

Activities:

Choose an activity you like and use it in addition or as a substitute to your existing exercise program.

Tennis	Cycling
Swimming	Hiking
Basketball	Racquetball
Squash	Ice skating
Roller skating	In-line skating
Volleyball	Golf (walk)
Softball	Frisbee
Paddle tennis	Smash ball

How about playing catch with your kids?

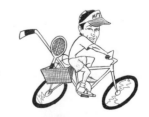

Maybe there is an activity you like that I didn't mention. Whatever it is, go for it. The idea is to *get your body moving.* It's up to you.

Self-Awareness Quiz

1 How much physical exercise are you getting each week?

daily yoga, walks

2 Are you consuming healthy foods? _trying to_

3 How many hours of sleep are you getting each night?

_8_

4 What methods are you using to manage stress?

_ha ha_

Weekly Appointments

☐ Appointment #1

- ◆ Do ___ toe raises.
- ◆ Do ___ curls.
- ◆ Do ___ push-ups.
- ◆ Do ___ sit-ups.
- ◆ Do ___ lunges.
- ◆ Walk ___ minutes.
  CHALLENGE: ___ intervals of ___ seconds each.
- ◆ Stretch.

☐ Appointment #2

- ◆ Do ___ toe raises.
- ◆ Do ___ curls.
- ◆ Do ___ push-ups.
- ◆ Do ___ sit-ups.
- ◆ Do ___ lunges.
- ◆ Walk ___ minutes.
  CHALLENGE: ___ intervals of ___ seconds each.
- ◆ Stretch.

☐ Appointment #3

- ◆ Do ___ toe raises.
- ◆ Do ___ curls.
- ◆ Do ___ push-ups.
- ◆ Do ___ sit-ups.
- ◆ Do ___ lunges.
- ◆ Walk ___ minutes.
  CHALLENGE: ___ intervals of ___ seconds each.

Weekly Appointments

☐ Appointment #1

- ♦ Do ___ toe raises.
- ♦ Do ___ curls.
- ♦ Do ___ push-ups.
- ♦ Do ___ sit-ups.
- ♦ Do ___ lunges.
- ♦ Walk ___ minutes.
  CHALLENGE: ___ intervals of ___ seconds each.
- ♦ Stretch.

☐ Appointment #2

- ♦ Do ___ toe raises.
- ♦ Do ___ curls.
- ♦ Do ___ push-ups.
- ♦ Do ___ sit-ups.
- ♦ Do ___ lunges.
- ♦ Walk ___ minutes.
  CHALLENGE: ___ intervals of ___ seconds each.
- ♦ Stretch.

☐ Appointment #3

- ♦ Do ___ toe raises.
- ♦ Do ___ curls.
- ♦ Do ___ push-ups.
- ♦ Do ___ sit-ups.
- ♦ Do ___ lunges.
- ♦ Walk ___ minutes.
  CHALLENGE: ___ intervals of ___ seconds each.

Weekly Appointments

☐ Appointment #1

- Do ___ toe raises.
- Do ___ curls.
- Do ___ push-ups.
- Do ___ sit-ups.
- Do ___ lunges.
- Walk ___ minutes.
  CHALLENGE: ___ intervals of ___ seconds each.
- Stretch.

☐ Appointment #2

- Do ___ toe raises.
- Do ___ curls.
- Do ___ push-ups.
- Do ___ sit-ups.
- Do ___ lunges.
- Walk ___ minutes.
  CHALLENGE: ___ intervals of ___ seconds each.
- Stretch.

☐ Appointment #3

- Do ___ toe raises.
- Do ___ curls.
- Do ___ push-ups.
- Do ___ sit-ups.
- Do ___ lunges.
- Walk ___ minutes.
  CHALLENGE: ___ intervals of ___ seconds each.

Weekly Appointments

☐ Appointment #1

- ◆ Do ___ toe raises.
- ◆ Do ___ curls.
- ◆ Do ___ push-ups.
- ◆ Do ___ sit-ups.
- ◆ Do ___ lunges.
- ◆ Walk ___ minutes.
  CHALLENGE: ___ intervals of ___ seconds each.
- ◆ Stretch.

☐ Appointment #2

- ◆ Do ___ toe raises.
- ◆ Do ___ curls.
- ◆ Do ___ push-ups.
- ◆ Do ___ sit-ups.
- ◆ Do ___ lunges.
- ◆ Walk ___ minutes.
  CHALLENGE: ___ intervals of ___ seconds each.
- ◆ Stretch.

☐ Appointment #3

- ◆ Do ___ toe raises.
- ◆ Do ___ curls.
- ◆ Do ___ push-ups.
- ◆ Do ___ sit-ups.
- ◆ Do ___ lunges.
- ◆ Walk ___ minutes.
  CHALLENGE: ___ intervals of ___ seconds each.

Food Diary

Keep *My Personal Trainer* by your side for 3 consecutive days this week. Record everything you eat or drink. Specify the amounts eaten and bracket the foods consumed at one sitting. (See the Sample Day below.) This will help you become aware or your eating habits.

Sample Day	Day One
Upon arising [glass of water]	
Breakfast [2 slices of toast with butter, 2 cups of coffee with cream and sugar, glass of orange juice]	
Mid-morning snack [muffin, banana, mint tea]	
[glass of water]	
[another glass of water]	
Lunch [tuna sandwich with lettuce & tomato, glass of milk, medium apple]	
Midafternoon Snack [cheese and crackers, glass of water]	
Dinner [2 pork chops, ear of corn, mashed potatoes, 1 scoop ice cream, coffee]	
Late night snack [popcorn]	
Bedtime [glass of water]	

Day Two	Day Three

Compare the above to Duf's Cantina (pg. 130). Any room for improvement? Listen to your body and eat accordingly.

Lunch Comparison

Compare the two lunches. Where do you stand?

Junk Lunch			Quality Lunch		
Food (g)	Calories	Fat	Food (g)	Calories	Fat
Cheeseburger (¼ pound)	660	38	Turkey w/Swiss (whole wheat)	375	11
Fries (medium)	370	20	Mustard	2	0
			Mayo	109	11
Chocolate shake (medium)	410	11	Salad	265	9
			Milk (2%)	150	5
Apple pie	320	14	Fruit (apple)	100	0
Total	1,760	83g	Total	1,001	36g
			Pasta (still hungry!)	250	1
			Total	1,251	37g

Let's Do Lunch—Part I

Take me to lunch every day this week and write down what you eat.
Make a conscious effort to improve the quality of your lunches.

Monday

_____

_____

_____

_____

Tuesday

_____

_____

_____

Wednesday

_____

_____

_____

Thursday

_____

_____

_____

_____

Friday

_____

_____

_____

Saturday

_____

_____

Sunday

_____

_____

Let's Do Lunch—Part II

Take me to lunch every day this week and write down what you eat. Make a conscious effort to improve the quality of your lunches.

Monday

_____

_____

_____

Tuesday

_____

_____

_____

Wednesday

_____

_____

_____

Thursday

_____

_____

_____

Friday

_____

_____

_____

Saturday

_____

_____

_____

Sunday

_____

_____

_____

Compare Part One to Part Two.

Any improvement?

Sleep Chart

This week keep a sleep chart. How many hours are you getting each night? Keep a bar graph.

Hours of Sleep

| 12 |
| 11 |
| 10 |
| 9 |
| 8 |
| 7 |
| 6 |
| 5 |
| 4 |
| 3 |
| 2 |
| 1 |

Mon   Tues   Wed   Thurs   Fri   Sat   Sun

Hours of Sleep

| 12 |
| 11 |
| 10 |
| 9 |
| 8 |
| 7 |
| 6 |
| 5 |
| 4 |
| 3 |
| 2 |
| 1 |

Mon   Tues   Wed   Thurs   Fri   Sat   Sun

About the Authors

John Duffy has been a personal trainer for the past 10 years. His clients have included celebrities, businessmen and women, housewives, weekend warriors, world-class athletes, and children. Mr. Duffy, a graduate of UCLA, is a Doctor of Chiropractic and currently attends medical school.

Megan Williams is a client and friend of John Duffy. Ms. Williams is a founder of Tripod, a national program for deaf children and their families. The mother of two children, she is also a documentary film and TV producer. Megan is the recipient of numerous awards, including an Oscar nomination and the Columbia Dupont Journalism Award.

Index

foot exercise, 105
forearm exercises, 12
fruits, 132

gastrocs, 97
gluteus maximus, 67
goals, fitness, 2, 107, 117
grocery shopping, 131-134
grooming, 89

hamstrings, 67
heart muscle, 119
injury prevention, 61, 124
interval walking, 15

jet lag, 106
jogging, 141
Journal of the American Medical Association, 18
jump roping, 141
junk food, 49, 77, 133

leg care, 56
leg exercise, 61
leg muscles, 61, 67, 97
lunch, 130, 151-153
lunges, 61, 67

magnesium, 28
massage, self, 67, 139-140
maximum heart rate, 117, 120
meal planning, 24-25, 28-29, 32-33, 130-136
metabolism, 102
morning stretch, 125
mouth care, 21, 89
muscle cramp, 98

muscle soreness, 49, 67
muscles,
    abdominals, 23
    arm, 41, 79
    calf, 97
    chest, 41
    facial, 8, 68
    leg, 5, 61, 97
    stomach, 23
    thigh, 67

napping, 138-139
nutrition, 24-25, 28-29, 32-33, 48, 77, 130-136

pectorals, 41
pollution, 52
posture, 23, 41, 71, 73
potassium, 28
practice, 2-3
protein, 132-133
push-ups, 41-43, 45

quadriceps, 67

recovery breathing, 122-123
recovery period, 15
relaxation, 44, 69, 83, 123, 138-139
rest, 44-45, 138-139
resting heart rate, 117, 119-120
rowing machines, 141

S.A.I.D. principle, 118
self-awareness quiz, 143
self-massage, 67, 139-140
shoes, choosing, 5

vitamins, 48

walking,
    benefits of, 5, 18
    choosing routes, 52
    interval, 15
water, 10, 13, 57

weight lifting, 141
weight loss, 32, 136, 137-138
weight management, 32-33
weights, 79
wound treatment, 88

yoga, 141